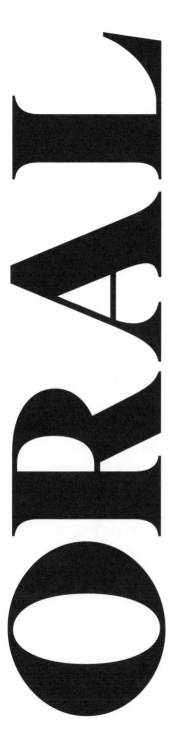

"As someone I have known and trusted for years, Jessica Lederhausen and I are aligned in our lifestyle-based approach to sustainable wellness. Through her unique lens as a Swedish-born dentist, public health advocate and 'lagom' (balance) coach, she makes the crucial connection between oral health and systemic health that is grounded in science, with actionable steps optimize our health and well-being. Highly recommended!"
— Dean Ornish, MD

"This book is more than just a guide; it's a catalyst for change in how we perceive and approach oral health. Jessica's passion for the subject is palpable on every page, making Oral not only informative but also deeply inspiring. It's a must-read for anyone dedicated to fostering a healthier, more balanced lifestyle, starting from the mouth, the gateway to our overall well-being."
— Avanti Kumar Singh, MD

"Jessica Lederhausen's book, Oral, is a masterful exploration of health pillars like nutrition, sleep, movement, and breathing. With elegance, she simplifies complex medical concepts, making them easily understandable. Dr. Lederhausen unveils the crucial link between oral health and overall well-being. The book not only elucidates these ideas but also provides practical solutions, offering a valuable guide to forming habits that lay the foundation for optimal health."
— Maria Sokolina, DDS

ORAL

Munhälsa

[*moon-hel-sah*]

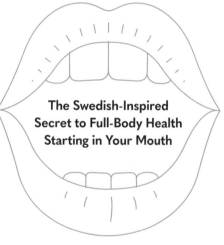

The Swedish-Inspired
Secret to Full-Body Health
Starting in Your Mouth

Jessica Lederhausen

DDS MPH

First published in 2024 by Jessica Lederhausen,
in partnership with Whitefox Publishing

www.wearewhitefox.com

ISBN 9781916797352
Also available as an eBook
ISBN 9781915635457

Designed and typeset by Louise Evans
Cover design by Louise Evans
Project management by whitefox
Author photo on back cover by Johnny Castle

thelagommethod.com
@jessicalederhausen

To Mats, Rebecca, Alexandra,
Theodore and Rosanna

DISCLAIMER

This book is not meant to be taken as medical advice or treatment, and it must not be interpreted that way. It's intended to assist you in making knowledgeable decisions regarding your overall health.

There can be no guarantees that following my advice will help you on your path to better health, therefore even if it proves to be helpful, it is still suggested that you consult a skilled physician for any medical issues, to receive treatment and/or an assessment. Any use of the information in this book is made on the reader's good judgment and is the reader's sole responsibility. Do not stop or change any prescription medications without the guidance and advice of your physician.

Dr. Jessica Lederhausen does not perform dental procedures and neither does she treat nor identify ailments or disorders. People should seek out diagnoses and take responsibility for any essential medical actions if they require dental or medical monitoring, diagnosis, and/or potential treatment.

ACKNOWLEDGMENTS

To Mats, my husband and life partner, whom I love more every day, every week, and every year we spend together. I really appreciate your patience in listening to me talking for the past almost 40 years (who's counting!) about the importance of the mouth and oral health as part of overall health. I also love that we both share an endless curiosity and excitement for exploring new ideas and new habits (sometimes crazy) in the interest of finding ways to be happier and healthier. Thank you for all the encouragement and support along the way to help me turn these ideas into a book.

Thank you to all my wonderful, loving, and amazing children who keep impressing me with your kindness, knowledge, and wisdom. I love you all so much. Rebecca, Alexandra, Theodore, and Rosanna.

Thank you to my sons-in-law and all my grandchildren for being just who you are and showing so much love and kindness to [*mormor/farmor*] Jessica. A large part of my own motivation behind trying to live these ideas is that I so very much want to experience the young men and women you will turn out to be.

A big thank you to my parents, Pyan and Ralph Posener, who obviously were there from the beginning and have always encouraged me to be as committed to my roots as to my wings.

Thank you to my siblings and their children for adding both challenge and support to my life.

To my father-in-law, Palle, who has inspired me with his passion, perseverance, and endless belief in the art of the possible.

I am also lucky and grateful to be surrounded by so many friends that keep inspiring me to learn more and stay curious, particularly in and around the area of health, habits, happiness, and family;

Suzanne Muchin, Dean Ornish MD, Mark Hyman MD, Avanti Kumar-Singh MD, Kjell Enhager, Mikael Zimmerman DDS, PhD, Fabrice Braunrot, Michael and Lisa Bronner, Annika Engel MD, Anders Olsson, Ellie Philips DDS, Yvonne Freund-Levi MD, PhD, Marina Klagsbrun, Helen Alfredsson, Catty Terling DDS, PhD, Avy and Marcie Stein, Judi and Steve Fader, Dov and Maria Seidman, Jill and Eric Becker, Larry and Margot Lessans, Carmela and Martin Gerson-Fuchs, Michel and Helen Gordin, Lotta Falck, Andrea and Barry Sidorow MD, Ann-Therese and Eli Hyman, Norin Guy, Gabriella Sellman, Annika Valdiserri, Alexandra Montgomery, Tony and Laura Tjan, Brian Bacon, Åsa and Anders Söderlund.

I would also like to express my special thanks to the group of people that helped me make this book come to life: Isabelle White, Rea Frey, Tracy Glass, and Annabel Wright with Whitefox Publishing.

A group hug to my wonderful, inspiring, uplifting, curious Circle friends, with whom I have had the honor and privilege to prototype many of these ideas in a virtual (and sometimes live) setting. Your feedback, reactions, and subsequent discussions have been instrumental in shaping the views I share in this book. And finally, to you holding this book, it is my hope that the ideas outlined here can act as a catalyst for creating new habits that will help you reach your goals and aspirations on your way toward becoming who you want to be.

Motivation is what gets you started.

Habit is what keeps you going.

– Jim Rohn

CONTENTS

FOREWORD

In medical school our mouth and teeth were somehow not on the curriculum. While it is obvious that doctors and dentists need different skill sets, what was not so obvious then was just how important our oral health is to our overall health. It shouldn't be surprising, as our body is one whole interconnected system. Mounting research has linked our oral health, and our oral microbiome, to a wide range of health conditions, from heart disease to dementia, from diabetes to colon cancer and even our risk of respiratory infections and asthma. It even impacts pregnancy outcomes including pre-term labor and low birthweight. But how are these things connected? Poor dental health creates inflammation not just in the mouth but throughout the body, and inflammation is the single biggest driver of chronic disease and aging itself. The mouth, and your overall dental health, are critical components of our overall health. Optimizing your oral health involves far more than just brushing your teeth twice a day.

As Jessica Lederhausen makes clear in this groundbreaking book, our dental health is impacted by much more than our oral hygiene. What we eat, how we move, sleep and manage stress are all essential in maintaining dental health, which then supports the rest of our body in staying healthy.

Our diet plays an outsized role in our dental health. I first learned about this by reading the works of Weston Price, a dentist at the turn of the last century who traveled the world with a notebook and a camera documenting the changing mouth structure, dental health, and chronic disease that occurred when hunter-gatherer tribes adopted a Western diet. Those tribes had perfect teeth and no cavities even though they never saw a dentist or orthodontist.

I recently had the chance to visit Africa and see the skulls of gorillas, elephants, giraffes, lions, and other mammals. What struck me was their perfect teeth. No cavities, no missing teeth, no need for orthodontics. What has changed more than anything is our diet from a whole food, nutrient, and fiber-dense diet to a highly processed, low-fiber diet. This has not only affected our risk of chronic diseases but profoundly impacted our dental health. I also visited a Maasai tribe who historically lived on the meat, milk, and blood of their cows. On being greeted into their village I was shocked to see that many had horrible teeth: rotted and misshapen and out of place. They were in desperate need of an orthodontist and a dentist. Then I realized what had been happening. In the late afternoon, just as it did every afternoon, in a village with no electricity or running water, the Coca Cola truck drove into their village and within minutes the entire truck, filled with soda, was emptied by the Maasai.

Thankfully, science is now recognizing the importance and relationship between our oral health and our overall health and aging. *Oral* is a powerful roadmap to upgrade your health by addressing dental health. In this step-by-step guide you will earn everything you need to take care of this oft neglected part of our body and improve your overall health.

— **Mark Hyman, MD**
Author of *Young Forever*
Founder and Senior Advisor, Cleveland Clinic Center
for Functional Medicine

INTRODUCTION: WHO I AM AND WHY THIS BOOK

I'm here to help you find new, easier, permanently effective ways to better your own health and create a balanced lifestyle. And the first thing you need to do in order to achieve that goal is, as I used to say when I was seeing my own dental patients in Sweden, "Open wide."

Why? Because, as I've come to realize over the course of a long career, everything in your body is connected, and the mouth is the body part where it all begins. The microorganisms (bacteria, viruses, and fungi) that live in the various parts of your body (mainly your gut) are all related to and influenced by those that inhabit your mouth.

It seems obvious, doesn't it? But for a long time, it wasn't—to me or to many of my fellow practitioners. But you're a dentist, you say; how could it have taken you so long to understand?

Truth be told, dentists aren't trained to think about whole body health in relation to the mouth; conversely, doctors aren't trained to see dental health as a first step to overall well-being.

Hippocrates, "the father of medicine," wrote about having treated (and cured) his patients using tooth extraction, tooth ointment, and oral tissue cauterization.

Once I began digging deeper into this connection, even with my professional background I found myself at times confused and overwhelmed by the amount of health advice out there, as well as by the fact that so much of it seems so complicated and extreme. There was a lot of information available, but not a lot that I could actually use and apply to my daily life in a practical, actionable way. As a dentist, as a former athlete, as a mother, and as a grandmother, I've always wanted a more holistic approach based on sustainable habits to which I can commit—a how-to manual for how to live my best and healthiest life. So, based on what I've learned from my extensive research as well as my personal health issues, that's exactly what I'm going to provide for you.

In addition to being a dentist and having a master's degree in public health, I'm a certified life coach and Tiny Habits coach, and a former professional golfer. I attended dental school, practiced dentistry, and played competitive golf while having four children in my native Sweden, before moving to the United States with my husband when I was in my mid-thirties. I'm telling you all this so that you'll understand why everyone who knows me says that I am a woman on a mission. My most defining quality is that I'm always asking why and (probably because of my background as a professional athlete) trying to improve my game.

As a dentist in Sweden and then working as a public health advocate in Chicago, I have always looked for ways to optimize my health and the health of those around me. Now, as a health coach, my mission is to help people set and achieve their own health goals.

Over the past years, as research has taught us more and more about how everything in the body is connected, I started to realize I had missed the crucial role dental health plays in good overall health throughout life.

MY OWN WAKE-UP CALL

Obviously, I don't know exactly why you decided to read my book, but I'm guessing that you have a reason for wanting to make some changes in the way you've been tending to your own health. Maybe a healthcare professional has told you it's time to start doing something different, or maybe you've had a health scare that prompted you to change things up.

As a dentist, I am passionate about oral hygiene. I brush my teeth twice a day. I floss carefully on a regular basis. I get biannual checkups with my own dentist. Taking care of my mouth has always been part of the way I care for my body. And I thought I had it covered.

But sometimes life throws you a curveball. My lower front teeth have had receding gums for years. Cosmetically, it didn't bother me, and I believed I had the problem under control—until, on one of my biannual visits, my wonderful dentist, whom I love and trust, told me that I should "probably see a specialist." For which read periodontist, a dentist who specializes in treating gum disease, often by making a tiny incision and lifting the gum back along the root of the tooth, exposing less of the tooth. A process sometimes referred to by the patient—me—as "cutting up my gums."

My brain began to spin. I knew exactly what the dentist was telling me, and I really wanted no part of it. Does anyone ever really *want* to have surgery, no matter how "minor" it might be? Nevertheless, after dragging my feet for a while, I finally made the appointment. The periodontist, like my dentist, was very nice and very persuasive, and I almost found myself convinced. But I *really* didn't want to have surgery. Surely, I thought, there must be some other way to deal with my receding gums.

As I was walking back home, visions of scalpels swirling around in my head, I had a great big "aha" moment. I realized that no one—not my dentist and not the oral surgeon—had even tried to talk to me about the underlying cause of the problem. Surely until I had that information, surgery would be nothing more than a band-aid solution. It wouldn't treat or even prevent the recurrence of whatever had caused the problem in the first place. Perhaps if I could discover the cause, I might be able to find a better way to heal my gums, or at least stop the deteriorating health in my mouth. It was certainly worth a try. Anything to escape those scalpels.

So, I got to work researching. I was open to trying anything that would help me avoid surgery. Searching for answers helped me discover what I had always known but often forgot. That causes and effects are not the same thing. Too often when we think about health we feel inclined to attack the effect. Not the cause. My problem was the receding gums. But what was the underlying cause of this problem? Clearly, having surgery would restore the gums but wouldn't fix what was causing the problem in the first place. The research I read, particularly around microbiome, helped me more plainly see that it was likely an imbalance in my microbiome in my mouth that was contributing to the receding gums. I ultimately explored different ways of both testing and rebalancing the health of my oral microbiome, and I believe that partly helped me avoid surgery. Subsequently I also learned other ways to contribute to a healthier mouth, and the four pillars in Part 2 of this book form what I now believe are the most important foundation for anyone wanting a healthier and happier life.

I don't want to suggest that you shouldn't have surgery under any circumstances, periodontal or otherwise, if that turns out to be the best option for you. But I am challenging you to look for the root cause of your problem so that you clearly understand all your options. And, of course, the solution shouldn't be worse than the problem. The cure can't be worse than the disease.

My philosophy around health is very much centered around the concept of *lagom*:

> *In Sweden, the concept of* lagom—*often translated as "moderation"—is part of the cultural currency. It's used to describe a situation that is not too much, not too little, but just right for you.*

This is, of course, nothing new. We might also refer to this as the Goldilocks Principle, a term used to refer to the human inclination to seek what is "just the right amount" of something. This is what I'm always searching for when I'm trying to make changes that will improve my own overall health. And it's the basis for what I'm going to be talking about here.

A HOLISTIC APPROACH

The key lies in understanding and, if necessary, adjusting the basics—what you do, often without even being aware of it—every day as you go about living your life. My approach to optimizing health is based on what I call my four pillars of health: eating, sleeping, breathing, and moving both your body and your mind. And I firmly believe that these principles run through all aspects of our general well-being in a way that is too often ignored.

For instance, has your dentist ever asked you about your overall health habits? Has your doctor ever asked about your oral health?

Dentistry and medicine split into two subspecialties in the 1900s. Unfortunately doing that caused us to think about different parts of the body as being unrelated to one another. The teeth in particular came to be seen as disconnected from the rest of the body. But, of course, they are not. And this is now starting to be recognized. The FDI (World Dental Federation) state on their website that they work with their members "to raise awareness about the importance of good oral health and its vital role in securing overall health and well-being. We are dedicated," they say, "to safeguarding the health of people worldwide through the improved prevention, treatment, and control of oral diseases."

I'll be very curious to see how (or if) the education and practice of dentistry changes in the future, because I believe that dentists need to work more closely with doctors in order to give patients the attention and care they need. Oral health includes the ability to speak, smile, smell, taste, touch, chew, swallow, and convey a range of emotions through facial expressions with confidence and without pain, discomfort, or disease of the craniofacial complex.

One of the problems with our modern system of healthcare in general is that, as medicine has become more and more specialized, every specialist tends to look at the problem being presented from their particular point of view—which is why you've probably heard someone say, "Well, they are a surgeon, so of course they're going to tell you that you need an operation." It's the medical equivalent of not being able to see the forest for the trees.

As I took a deep dive into my own oral health situation, I came upon a ton of information that was new to me. In fact, research is making it increasingly clear that we must understand the mouth as the gateway to the entire body. An unhealthy mouth is associated with an increased risk for a wide variety of health issues, including

Alzheimer's, diabetes, cardiovascular disease, and adverse pregnancy outcomes. In short, you can't be truly healthy without a healthy mouth.

Here's one small example. If you've ever had a problem with your heart, you may be advised to take antibiotics before visiting your dentist. That's because people with certain heart conditions are at risk for developing endocarditis, a serious heart infection, from the bacteria in their mouth. But, as you'll discover over the course of this book, that's really just the tip of the iceberg—the one connection between oral and overall health that many of us already know enough to look out for—and there are so many others.

Early in my career as a dentist, I became more and more interested in barriers to health. In Sweden, we enjoy a generous healthcare system which includes free dental care for anyone up to age 23. And yet some people took far greater advantage of the healthcare available, while others did not, only to later discover serious health problems in their mouths. Why was this? I became so fascinated by this question that my colleagues encouraged me to enter a Ph.D. program exploring barriers to health.

The team I had joined was designing mobile care units in the belief that, by bringing the care to the patients, we would reduce barriers to health such as inconvenience, fear, and cultural norms, among others. While my move to the United States in 1999 prevented me from completing this research, I saw enough data to convince me of the need to look at healthcare in a more holistic way. Our health habits are very much influenced by our social, psychological, and physical environment. Therefore, when I think about helping anyone (myself included) to change a habit, I try to consider practicalities as much as scientific and technical issues. At the end of the day, a good habit only stays with you if you make it easy enough, balancing what is theoretically optimal with what is practically doable. Which, of course, goes back to the concept of *lagom*.

ONE SMALL STEP AT A TIME

Other than a simple lack of knowledge, one major roadblock to achieving optimal health is that, as with virtually everything in life, people typically focus on the outcome rather than the process. But if you want to be happy, you can't just focus on happiness. Similarly, if you want to be healthy, you can't just focus on health. Instead, I believe, you need to focus on the *actions* that produce health.

As an example, taken from my career as a golfer, you can't improve your score by focusing on lowering your score. One of the most important lessons I learned from my coaches is that, in trying to improve my game, I needed to determine what long-term result I was seeking, then break that down into smaller steps. Where could I improve? Was it my short game? Consistency in my tee shots? Was I in the right mindset? Did I need to adjust my physical training? You get it. Once I'd figured that out, I could begin to improve each element by implementing practice habits that would help me reach each goal. The end result fulfilled my aspiration for a lower overall score. It's a process. One step at a time.

The problem is that when it comes to health—and particularly mouth health—we may not even realize there's a problem until it becomes a crisis, and most of us don't know how to begin to fix it. I certainly didn't when I began to research alternatives to oral surgery. And it is complicated, because of course all of our systems and organs are so interconnected. I am hoping that, by writing this book, I can share what I have learned and hopefully make it easy to understand for others and even easier to integrate into your own daily habits.

"Health" is a simple word that conveys a big idea. It can seem like such a big mountain to climb that you don't even want to put your hiking boots on. In *Oral*, the path to improved health begins in the mouth and is divided into smaller steps.

PART

1

EVERYTHING
IS
CONNECTED

CHAPTER 1

Many of us clean our teeth in front of the mirror every day. But when was the last time you took a really good, close look at your mouth?

OPEN WIDE

[*Öppna upp*]

Your mouth (or oral cavity) starts at the lips and ends where the mouth meets the throat. It includes the teeth, tongue, cheeks, gums, salivary glands, the hard and soft palates, and the tonsils. It is the beginning of the aerodigestive tract, which links the upper part of the digestive tract (the esophagus, stomach, and the first part of the small intestine) to the organs and tissues of the respiratory tract, including the nose, the nasal cavity, and the throat.

In other words, there's a lot going on in your mouth. And from the color of your gums to the texture of your tongue, your mouth has got a lot to tell you—without even saying a word.

YOUR ORAL MICROBIOME

In addition to all the parts of the oral cavity you can see in the illustration opposite, there's a lot more to the picture that you can't see. You may never have heard the term "microbiome." Or, if you have, it was probably in reference to the bacteria and other microbes living in your gut. But your mouth is also home to somewhere between 700 and 900 different species of bacteria, viruses, and fungi, totaling millions of individual organisms—the oral microbiome. The composition of the microbiome is unique to each individual person in much the same way that each person's DNA is unique.

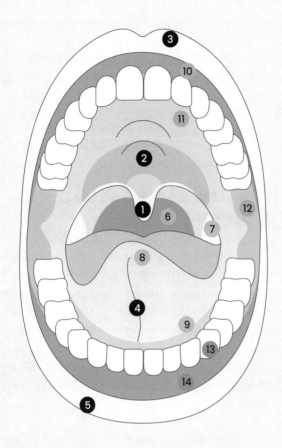

1. Uvula
2. Soft palate
3. Upper lip
4. Lingual frenulum
   (underside of tongue)
5. Lower lip

● Habitat 1
6. Throat
7. Palatine tonsil
8. Tongue
9. Salivary duct orifices

● Habitat 2
10. Gums (gingivae)
11. Hard palate
12. Buccal mucosa
    (inside the cheek)

● Habitat 3
13. Supragingival plaque
    (above the gums)

● Habitat 4
14. Subgingival plaque
    (below the gums)

Most of us grew up believing that all bacteria are bad and that in order to be healthy we need to get rid of them—wipe them out of our system entirely. We've been told that bacteria in our mouth can cause cavities, gum disease, and bad breath, all of which is true—up to a point. But it isn't the whole story. In fact, our mouths are home to all sorts of microbes. What we really need to do is not strip it of *all* its tiny inhabitants, but to maintain a healthy balance of all the different types.

ORAL HOMEOSTASIS (BALANCE)

Homeostasis refers both to the state of maintaining equilibrium among your physiological and biological systems (in this case, the bacteria in your mouth) and the process of achieving that stability by adjusting to changing conditions. Different parts of your mouth are home to different habitats (colonies) of various bacteria, and the goal is to maximize the *variety*—or, in other words, to maintain a diverse oral microbiome, aka "microbiota." It's all about balance. Oral homeostasis is achieved and maintained by keeping a healthy relationship between your saliva and the organisms in your oral microbiome.

Saliva is a watery liquid produced by the salivary glands in the mouth. The saliva contains electrolytes, including phosphates, sodium, potassium, magnesium, calcium, and bicarbonates, as well as enzymes and proteins. Together these provide lubrication for chewing and swallowing, aid in digestion, wash away debris, and help prevent bacterial overgrowth by balancing the pH, as well as protecting against tooth erosion, and even working as a line of defense against infections in your mouth. We produce a remarkable 1 to 1.5 liters of saliva per day.

SALIVA

1 **ELECTROLYTES:** Phosphates, sodium, potassium, magnesium, and calcium (minerals) help maintain the balance of fluids in the mouth and are essential for normal cell function and nerve transmission.

2 **BICARBONATES:** These help maintain the pH balance in the mouth by acting as a buffer, reducing acidity, which protects the teeth from erosion.

3 **ENZYMES:** Present in saliva, these aid in the breakdown of carbohydrates and fats during digestion.

4 **IMMUNOGLOBULINS:** Also known as antibodies, these are part of the immune system's defense mechanism. They help neutralize harmful bacteria and viruses in the mouth, protecting against infections and maintaining oral health.

Microbiota, including bacteria, fungi, and viruses, are present in the mouth in various combinations and quantities that create the oral microbiome. The microbiota can change over time due to the host's (your) changes in circumstances, such as the use of antimicrobial products or probiotics or lack of sleep.

THE FACTS

- Nearly half (46 percent) of all adults aged 30 years or older show signs of gum disease; severe gum disease affects about 9 percent of adults.

- Among adults aged 20 and older, about 90 percent have had at least one cavity.

- One in four adults aged 20 to 64 currently has at least one untreated cavity.

HOW IT WORKS

The opposite of oral homeostasis is oral dysbiosis, which occurs when the bacteria in your mouth are out of balance, potentially leading to inflammation of the gums, periodontitis, and/or tooth decay. Whenever we eat or drink, we're interrupting homeostasis.

During homeostasis, there is a biofilm (the microbiome) covering areas in the mouth, such as teeth, tongue, chin and more, which acts like a protection shield.

Problems can occur when there is an imbalance of the microbiome, which happens when there is an overgrowth of pathogenic (disease-causing) bacteria within the biofilm. This can then lead to the accumulation of dental plaque on the teeth. Dental plaque is a soft, sticky film of bacteria and their byproducts. If dental plaque is not effectively removed through proper oral hygiene practices, it can mineralize and harden over time, forming dental calculus or tartar.

The acids in plaque eat away at your tooth enamel, eventually causing decay, and find their way under your gums to cause periodontal disease. In fact, dental plaque is one of the main causes of dental disease.

Saliva is one of our best natural defenses against the damage caused by plaque, because it contains calcium, phosphorous, fluoride, and other minerals that help to neutralize the acids in plaque and also repair the damage they do to the enamel on the surface of your teeth.

Streptococcus mutans is one type of bacteria living in your mouth, specifically in dental plaque, and *lactobacillus* is another. Both feed on sugars and other fermentable carbohydrates. When we eat any food, but especially sugary foods, these bacteria feed on it, multiply, and thrive. As they do, they excrete acid, which lowers the pH balance in your mouth. This acidic environment eats away at the tooth enamel. Then, under circumstances that we'll be discussing later in this book, your saliva either does or doesn't restore the pH balance in your mouth. If the saliva is not able to do what it's supposed to, the pH stays low and the acid continues to eat away at your teeth. Keep reading to find out in the chapters on the four pillars what you can do to ensure that your saliva is able to function the way it's supposed to.

PROTECT YOUR MOUTH TO PROTECT YOUR BODY

If saliva is your first line of defense against plaque, the oral cavity itself is your first line of defense against many diseases of the body. Because your mouth is the point of entry for the vast majority of everything that goes into your body, it stands to reason that a healthy body and a healthy mouth are inextricably connected.

STEPHAN'S CURVE: SINGLE SUGAR EXPOSURE

Robert M. Stephan found in his research in 1943—yes, that long ago!—that when you eat something sugary, you have a quick, intense reaction in your mouth by lowering the pH. This lower pH environment in the mouth means that you are now exposed to the possibility of tooth erosion. Luckily, you can also see in the graph below that the mouth returns to its normal levels in about 30 minutes. However, the point here is that your own "cleaning" system helps you after eating any food, but if you keep eating with a higher frequency, it might not keep up, and you will be exposing yourself to the risk of disease.

This is just part of the process, but at least it's something we know what to do about.

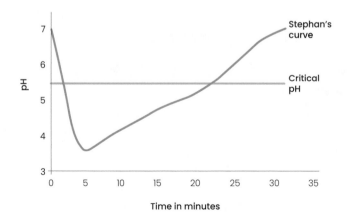

According to Cass Nelson-Dooley, author of *Heal Your Oral Microbiome*, we swallow about 140 billion bacteria every day, and 50 percent of the microbes in our gut are the same as those in our mouth. Clearly then, what starts in your mouth doesn't always stay in your mouth, which is why your oral health is intimately connected with and predictive of your overall health.

THE PROBLEM WITH BLEEDING GUMS

Bleeding gums may be an indication that you have periodontal disease, which can lead to bone loss in the jaws. But bleeding gums may also create problems outside your mouth, because they provide a way for the bacteria that have been living in your oral microbiome to escape and travel throughout your body via your bloodstream, causing or contributing to any number of diseases.

Even without periodontal disease, however, simple everyday behaviors, including brushing and/or flossing your teeth, can cause your gums to bleed, as can having a thorough cleaning at the dentist, which is why (as previously noted) people with some forms of cardiovascular disease are told to take an antibiotic before a dental visit.

You may have heard of leaky gut, which is what happens when the lining of the gut is damaged, allowing bacteria to "leak" out into other parts of the body where they don't belong. "Leaky mouth" is not an actual medical term, but—given the mouth's role as the gateway to the rest of the body—maybe it should be. Because this is exactly what happens when the oral cavity is damaged in a way that allows the bacteria in your oral microbiome to enter your bloodstream and cause disease in other parts of your body.

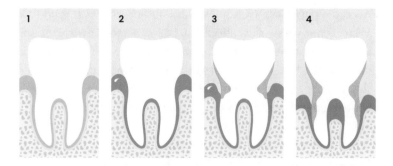

1 HEALTHY GUMS
- The crown is above the bone and gum lines.
- The root is under the bone and gum lines.
- The color of the gum is pinkish light red.

2 GINGIVITIS: INFLAMMATION OF THE GUMS
- Now the gum is swollen and has a red color. Typically it is shiny as well.
- Bone loss has not started.
- You might bleed when you brush your teeth. With a little more attention to cleaning for a couple of days, it goes away.

3 PERIODONTITIS
- The gum is swollen, red, and shiny.
- You might bleed when you brush your teeth. With some more attention to cleaning for a couple of days, it goes away.
- Bone loss has started but is not easily noticeable to the eye.

4 PERIODONTAL DISEASE
- This is worse, as we now see bone loss as well as gum loss.

Severe periodontal disease is estimated to affect around 1 billion people (approximately 19 percent of the global population).

In the following chapter, I'll be explaining how your body can affect your oral health and vice versa. And once you've become as intimately acquainted with your body as you now are with your mouth, it will be time to discuss what you can do to ensure that they are both as healthy as possible.

SUMMARY OF CHAPTER 1

1   Your mouth is more than just teeth and gums—it includes various components such as the tongue, cheeks, salivary glands, and tonsils.

2   The mouth is home to a diverse collection of bacteria, viruses, and fungi, collectively known as the oral microbiome. Maintaining a healthy balance of these microorganisms is crucial for oral health.

3   Saliva plays a vital role in oral health by providing lubrication, aiding digestion, washing away debris, and preventing bacterial overgrowth. It also helps balance pH, protects against tooth erosion, and acts as a defense against infections.

Western medicine tends to treat the body as a series of separate systems—such as the circulatory system, the digestive system, the nervous system, and so on. Therefore, when we have a health problem, we're generally instructed to see a specialist. But the fact is—and we know this instinctively—everything in our body is connected, and when something goes wrong, chances are that more than one of our systems is malfunctioning.

THE BODY CONNECTION

[*Koppling till kroppen*]

Modern life puts our bodies under a lot of stress. The air we breathe is full of pollutants; the food we eat can be overprocessed and lacking in nutrients; and the pressure of work can lead to high levels of stress and anxiety. The body, however, does its best to cope with whatever we throw its way. It learns to compensate for our bad habits. But by finding out more about how the body works and what it needs to stay healthy, we can help it to maintain a proper balance—and achieve that all-important state we discussed in the previous chapter: homeostasis.

THREE WAYS DISEASE CAN SPREAD FROM THE MOUTH TO OTHER BODY PARTS

1 INFECTION

Bacteria picked up during dental treatments or infections in the mouth can enter the bloodstream and travel throughout the body until they find a suitable place to settle, and, after some time, colonize and cause infection. An example known for decades is when bacteria travel and infect the inner lining of the heart valves, leading to endocarditis.

Aspiration of oral bacteria into the lungs can result in pneumonia, especially in people with reduced immune systems or lung function.

2 INJURY/TOXINS

Toxins can be produced by oral bacteria, such as those linked with gum disease or dental infections, as part of their regular metabolic processes. These toxins can be harmful to the surrounding oral tissues and may enter the bloodstream, allowing them to be transported to other parts of the body.

Examples of bacteria and toxins produced:

Porphyromonas gingivalis: This bacterium is linked to periodontal disease and can produce the toxin gingipains. These enzymes contribute to gum tissue breakdown and inflammation.

Streptococcus mutans: A primary bacterium contributing to dental caries (tooth decay). As a consequence of sugar metabolism, it creates acids, which can demineralize tooth enamel and lead to cavity development.

-----

3 ACUTE AND CHRONIC INFLAMMATION

Gum disease is often the source of the bacteria that cause the body to generate antibodies, which produce an acute or chronic inflammatory reaction.

INFLAMMATION AND THE IMMUNE SYSTEM

We are generally taught that inflammation is "not good"; it's a sign of some kind of injury or infection, and that is certainly true. But in most cases—if, for example, we've banged our thumb with a hammer, or we have a sore throat—inflammation is a sign that our immune system has mustered its army of defenders to resolve the problem. That's why, if you've been prescribed an antibiotic, you've also been told not to stop taking it until all the pills are used up, even if you're feeling better. What happens when you start taking an antibiotic is that all those little immune system soldiers go back to the barracks and relax, because they think the situation is under control. Therefore, if you stop taking your meds prematurely, before the infection is entirely irradicated, the infection will once more have free rein to do its dirty work.

But all that is true of what is generally called an acute problem—one that occurs, is resolved, and goes away. Chronic inflammation is a different story. When there is no acute cause such as infection or injury, and yet your body continues to deploy its immune system soldiers, you are suffering from chronic inflammation. This can result from an autoimmune disease that causes the body to attack its own healthy cells, such as lupus or rheumatoid arthritis; from continuous exposure to toxins; or from an acute infection that goes untreated.

The problem is that when you have chronic inflammation, your immune system is working overtime. Those little soldiers don't have a chance to go back to the barracks to rest and restore themselves. So, your immunity may actually be depleted. And if your immune cells are attacking your own cells rather than some foreign invader, they may also be damaging organs and tissues that were otherwise perfectly healthy. This can lead to you developing a potentially more serious, even life-threatening illness down the road.

REMEMBER TO LOOK IN YOUR MOUTH

In Traditional Chinese Medicine, or TCM, one of the most frequently used methods of diagnosis is to look at the tongue. The tongue is considered "the window to the body," and practitioners of TCM believe that its characteristics, such as shape, color, surface condition, and action, can reveal signs of disease or imbalance in other parts of the body.

As I keep saying, everything is connected, and what starts in your mouth can find its way into the rest of your body. When your mouth is healthy, you've eliminated at least one potential cause of infection in your body.

I wasn't surprised when a friend of mine told me this story: Her father had been "not himself" for some time. Very active by nature, he simply didn't have the energy to do all the things he normally enjoyed. But he'd consulted several doctors, and no one had been able to get to the source of the problem—until, that is, someone thought to look in his mouth, where, after three long months of ill-health, they finally found the infection!

Unfortunately, the mouth is too often the last place anyone looks when their body is out of whack. But the truth is that, if you can see signs of inflammation in your mouth, there's a pretty good chance that it's associated with inflammation elsewhere in your body.

We spend a lot of time talking about our gut, and most of us are aware that a happy gut translates to a happy body. But not so many of us understand the relationship between what's going on in our mouth and what's happening in our gut. That's unfortunate, because from the moment we enter the world, our birthing mother is passing on her microbiota, and as we take our first breath, microbiota from the bacteria-filled world is beginning to enter our body. Infants' first and essentially only real activity is eating. They can't control their extremities very well, but they can use their mouths. And whatever they ingest feeds both their oral and, via saliva, their gut microbiome. Anatomically, our gut and our mouth are not separate systems; they are one complete unit, so it should make perfect sense that the two microbiomes remain linked throughout our life.

THE HIGHWAY TO HEALTH IS A TWO-WAY STREET

We've already talked about the fact that what goes on in your mouth can affect your gut, but the reverse is also true. In many cases, the problems we see in the mouth are actually caused by problems that occur elsewhere in the body. Here are a few of the important links that have been established between the health of your mouth and the health of your body.

Cardiovascular disease: It has long been known that gum disease is linked to an increased risk for heart disease, and cardiovascular disease is the number-one cause of death in the United States.

Diabetes: This affects more than 37 million people in the United States, and more than one in four of them are unaware that they have the disease. Of these, 90 to 95 percent are type 2, which is often associated with lifestyle factors and insulin resistance. Periodontal disease can lead to or exacerbate diabetes due to inflammation, but, paradoxically, having high blood sugar levels associated with diabetes can also lead to gum disease. This happens because diabetes affects the quality of your saliva, which

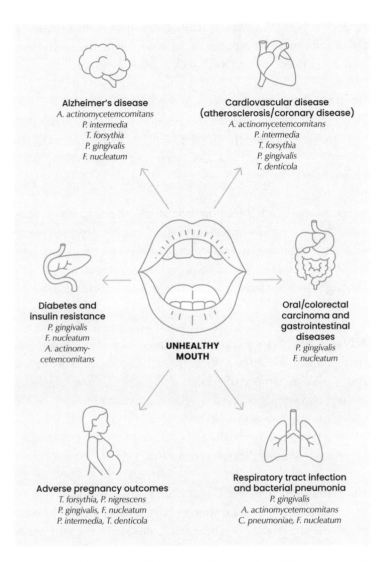

Alzheimer's disease
A. actinomycetemcomitans
P. intermedia
T. forsythia
P. gingivalis
F. nucleatum

Cardiovascular disease
(atherosclerosis/coronary disease)
A. actinomycetemcomitans
P. intermedia
T. forsythia
P. gingivalis
T. denticola

Diabetes and
insulin resistance
P. gingivalis
F. nucleatum
A. actinomy-
cetemcomitans

**UNHEALTHY
MOUTH**

Oral/colorectal
carcinoma and
gastrointestinal
diseases
P. gingivalis
F. nucleatum

Adverse pregnancy outcomes
T. forsythia, P. nigrescens
P. gingivalis, F. nucleatum
P. intermedia, T. denticola

Respiratory tract infection
and bacterial pneumonia
P. gingivalis
A. actinomycetemcomitans
C. pneumoniae, F. nucleatum

means that it is not as efficient at balancing the pH in your mouth to prevent gum disease. So, in the end, it's a vicious circle: gum disease increases blood glucose levels, which, in turn, increases your risk of developing gum disease.

Alzheimer's disease and dementia: There has been research that suggests a possible link between gum disease and Alzheimer's disease. While some studies have linked the bacteria

Porphyromonas gingivalis, a leading cause of gum disease, to the development or progression of Alzheimer's disease, further research is needed to establish a clear association.

Colorectal cancer: Scientists at the Harvard School of Public Health have found evidence that periodontal disease and loss of teeth may be linked to the development of colorectal cancer, the second leading cause of cancer death (after lung disease) in the United States.

Respiratory tract infection/bacterial pneumonia: Studies have shown that the mouth and the lung have similar microbiomes, suggesting a relationship between oral health and respiratory diseases, including pneumonia, asthma, and COPD, although the mechanisms through which this occurs are not yet well understood.

Adverse pregnancy outcomes: Pregnancy creates hormonal changes that can lead to an increase in inflammation in the mouth and the development of pregnancy gingivitis. Symptoms such as sore, swollen, and bleeding gums are common signs of this condition. Adverse outcomes may include complications such as preterm labor and low birthweight, although the full extent of the associated risks and outcomes can vary.

The Centers for Disease Control (CDC) has indicated that 60 to 75 percent of pregnant women have gingivitis. A lot of times there are changes in behavior while pregnant, such as eating habits and sleeping poorly. Pregnant women may also have more cavity-causing bacteria in their mouths, which puts them at risk of passing on these microorganisms to their children, both while giving birth and after. As we are constantly learning more, it's always a good idea to consult with your healthcare provider or dentist for the most up-to-date information and recommendations regarding oral health during pregnancy.

HOW YOUR MOUTH REFLECTS THE STATE OF YOUR GUT

A red or swollen tongue can be a sign of immune imbalance in the digestive system. Deficiency in folic acid and other B vitamins can also cause a swollen tongue.

Flat red patches on the gums and the inside of the cheeks can be a sign of vitamin B12 deficiency.

Oral candida or yeast infection is a sign of immune imbalance and may indicate a zinc deficiency resulting from poor digestive function.

Mouth ulcers, aphthous ulcers (aka canker sores), and red, inflamed gums can indicate digestive problems due to an immune imbalance in the gut.

White pus-filled lesions in the mouth are similar to those seen with Crohn's disease in the colon.

White lacy lesions in the mouth, sometimes accompanied by skin rashes and/or burning sensations in the mouth, may be related to having an autoimmune disease.

Burning mouth syndrome, as the name suggests, is the sensation of burning in the mouth that may also be accompanied by a loss of taste, dry mouth, and/or oral inflammation. This condition may suggest low levels of vitamins and minerals. However, it may also be a side effect of medications such as antidepressants.

In addition:

Leaky gut syndrome, which can be caused by an imbalance of bacteria, creates a permeability in your intestine that allows toxins to make their way back into your mouth and gums.

Gastroesophageal reflux disease (also known as GERD or acid reflux), which occurs when stomach acid moves back up through your digestive tract and your throat, can introduce destructive acids from your digestive system into your mouth, leading to tooth decay and an acidic environment in your saliva, not to mention halitosis.

Celiac disease is caused by an autoimmune response to gluten, and it often causes ulcers in the mouth.

Sjögren's disease, an immune response to cells that produce saliva, results in the breakdown of the salivary glands, reducing salivary flow. It can cause dry mouth (as well as dry eyes, skin rashes, joint pain, and numbness or tingling in the extremities) and increase the risk of tooth loss or decay.

Rheumatoid arthritis (RA) has been associated with an increased risk of gum disease, and sufferers are likely to experience more severe symptoms. One study has shown that people with RA are twice as likely to have gum disease as those who don't.

I'm writing this book because I wish we could include the mouth when we are looking at healthcare and when we treat patients with cancer, respiratory disease, ulcers, etc. Why not bring in a dentist to be on the caring team? Given everything that's being written and talked about regarding food as medicine, it's not hard to understand that what you eat affects not only your mouth but also your body. But it may be more of a stretch for you to appreciate how much your sleeping habits, the way you breathe, and even your mental attitude impact not only your body but also the health of your mouth. We'll be talking about all of that in the chapters that follow.

SUMMARY OF CHAPTER 2

1 Western medicine often treats the body as a collection of separate systems, but it's important to recognize that everything in the body is interconnected, and a health issue in one system can affect others.

2 There are three ways disease can spread from the mouth to other body parts: through infection, toxins produced by bacteria, and inflammation, with dental issues potentially affecting overall health.

3 The highway to health is a two-way street: what goes on in your mouth can affect your gut, but the reverse is also true. In many cases, the problems we see in the mouth are actually caused by problems that occur elsewhere in the body.

4 In Traditional Chinese Medicine, or TCM, the tongue is considered "the window to the body," and practitioners of TCM believe that its characteristics, such as shape, color, surface condition, and action, can reveal signs of disease or imbalance in other parts of the body.

CHAPTER 3

*What are habits? What do they do, and
how can I make new ones?*

HABITS

[*Vanor*]

The first thing I want you to understand is that we are all creatures of habit. Many of the things we do every day, we don't even think about. Maybe you automatically put your keys in the same place every day when you come home. That's a good habit: it ensures that you'll be able to find them when you go out again. Maybe when you get up in the morning you always make a pot of coffee and brush your teeth while it's brewing. Another good habit: not only are you cleaning your teeth, you're also guaranteeing that your coffee will be ready when it's time to sit down and have a peaceful moment with your morning brew as a reward.

But not every habit is "good." Maybe you mindlessly open the refrigerator and reach for a snack when you're bored. Or you automatically reach for the box of chocolates when you're upset.

BE AWARE OF YOUR HABITS

Even though the behaviors themselves may be automatic, we're still, on some level, aware of our habits, good and bad. Think about it: if you didn't know that you always put your keys in the dish by the front door, how would you automatically know where to retrieve them the next day?

My goal is to help you live your healthiest and, therefore, happiest, most rewarding life. And to do that, you need to become aware of the habits that may be holding you back; find new habits that can help you create momentum toward your aspirations. But don't worry! I'm not about to ask you to change your entire life. That would be self-defeating because you simply wouldn't do it. You'd probably just slam this book closed and proceed immediately to the refrigerator.

There are many small things you can do that will produce BIG results. Remember that "A journey of a thousand miles begins with a single step."*

HOW HABITS ARE FORMED

I have been interested in how habits are formed for as long as I can remember. I'm keen to learn how other people's habits are benefiting them and if I can incorporate them in my own life.

We form habits, most often unconsciously, via a psychological process called a "habit loop," which was first discovered by MIT researchers in the 1990s and later written about by the Pulitzer-Prize-winning journalist Charles Duhigg in his book *The Power of Habit: Why We Do What We Do in Life and Business.* A habit loop is composed of:

1 **THE CUE:** A trigger telling our brain to do a particular thing at a particular time. Since we're talking about oral health here, let's say that feeling it's time for bed triggers your brain to tell you it's time to brush your teeth.

2 **THE ROUTINE:** This is the behavior itself—in this case brushing your teeth. I have the toothbrush visible in my bathroom to help me remember what to do.

---

* "A journey of a thousand miles begins with a single step" is a common saying that originates from a Chinese proverb. The quotation is from Chapter 64 of the Dao De Jing, ascribed to Laozi, although it is also erroneously ascribed to his contemporary Confucius.

3 THE REWARD: The reward is something the brain likes, which helps it to remember to repeat the behavior. In this case, the reward would be feeling that you are properly prepared for bed.

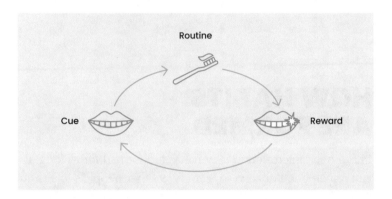

I'm very grateful to have had several wise teachers, including Stephen Covey, author of *The 7 Habits of Highly Effective People*; James Clear, author of *Atomic Habits*; and BJ Fogg, a behavioral scientist whose book, *Tiny Habits: The Small Changes that Change Everything*, inspired me to enroll in the program he created to become certified as a Tiny Habits coach.

I've learned a lot from these and other teachers, and I've distilled their wisdom into a personal philosophy and way of life that I hope and believe will work for you as well.

CREATING NEW HABITS, ONE STEP AT A TIME

Earlier in this book I talked about the fact that people tend to focus on their desired outcome (their aspiration), rather than on the process (the goals and habits that will help them achieve that outcome) that will take them there, and I compared it to my desire to improve my score as a professional golfer. But, as I pointed out, it's the process that will get you where you want to be. Your habits are your process. That's why they matter so much. They are the engine that will take you to your destination.

However, here is a very important point. Aspirations are as needed to enable habits as habits are to enable your aspirations. Aspirations are the WHY and habits are the WHAT, WHEN, WHERE, and HOW.

When you are creating new habits, make sure that they align with your overall aspiration.

LET'S GET STARTED

Take out a pencil and a piece of paper and make a list of all the things you want to achieve, accomplish, or that you aspire to do. I suspect once you get going, this list will be a long one. Some of these will be very serious aspirations, such as "I really want to become a lawyer," and some might be more along the lines of "I want to become a consistent runner."

Go over the list again and look more carefully. What is it that you really want to do?

Maybe the list is shorter now. Let's see if you can narrow it down to three or four things for now.

When you have those, it's time to get started.

Now that you have your aspirations written down, please look at the model I have created that I call the "4 C Habits for Creating Habits."

4 C HABITS FOR CREATING HABITS

CONNECT
It's important that whatever habit you are considering is connected to your overall life goals and aspirations. We don't set habits to master habits. They are a means to bigger ends. And if you don't see clearly how a new habit will lead you to where you truly want to be, you will not be successful in sticking to your new habit. Particularly when barriers and challenges surface. And they always do.

CURATE
Once you have a clear vision of why you want to start a new habit, it is time to curate your options on how to make it happen.

First, make sure you are not trying to move mountains or take on too big of a challenge. Start small. Be focused.

Second, try to integrate a new habit into the already existing patterns and rhythms of your life. Go with the grain instead of against it. It's also a good idea to "attach" a habit to something you are already doing on a regular basis. For example, meditating while going up in the elevator to your apartment; always parking your car farther away from the store or your office to get a few extra steps in, etc.

CREATE

When you are set on what new habits you want to commit to, consider the context of your life and make sure you remove all reasons to say no and make it as easy as you can to say yes.

For example: Do you have the right tools and equipment? Can you set prompts and reminders around the home or office and on your calendar? Perhaps my favorite: invite people you spend time with to practice the new habit with you. We often break promises to ourselves more than we break them to others. A strong supportive network is the best scaffolding for building new habits.

CELEBRATE

Make sure to celebrate the smallest wins and not be too hard on yourself. You see often how athletes fist-pump their small achievements. Those gestures are designed to cement and associate a good action with a positive outcome. The more you do that, the more that action will become automatic.

Cement (verb): To join or bond something firmly together, often used metaphorically to indicate the strengthening or solidifying of a relationship, agreement, or concept.

Here's an example taken from my own experience:

CONNECT

My aspiration is to be more present in everything I do, with closer proximity to joy.

CURATE

Since I have been dabbling in meditation for many years, I know if I had a more consistent meditation practice it would help me get closer to where I want to be. I also know that my morning routine is one of the few things in my life where I have the opportunity for less stress, fewer calls and interruptions, and less craziness. It's my time, and I can get even more out of it.

CREATE

While I am waiting for our fresh coffee to brew each morning, I will use the meditation app on my phone and sit in my favorite chair and meditate for two to four minutes. I will also set a repeating reminder every day on my calendar, so I don't forget.

CELEBRATE

Every day I meditate, I will celebrate with a pat on the shoulder and say, "Well done!"

The main purpose of writing this book is of course that I would like to be as helpful as possible to your overall health. As you also by now have realized, I am a firm believer that small changes can have big impacts, and the gateway to better health can best be found by examining and tweaking your daily habits.

Therefore, I have created worksheets at the end of each of the following chapters. These worksheets have been designed to guide you in exploring and creating new habits around the topic of each chapter, based on the 4 Cs.

LEARN TO WALK BEFORE YOU RUN

I remember watching my grandchild learn to take her first steps and reflecting on the difference between how children react to the process of learning compared to us older people. As she kept trying to take her first steps, she fell, repeatedly. Each time, we adults would cheer her on, saying things like, "Great! You're doing it!" And every time, she just smiled and tried again. It seemed to me then, and still seems to me now, that we need to adopt a similar attitude in our own process of trying new things. We may not have a cheering section watching us, but we can—and should—be our own cheerleaders. At what point in life do we stop believing that we can, and will, achieve whatever we aspire to, even if we take tiny steps and stumble along the way?

DOING "JUST ENOUGH"

I've already discussed the fact that the Swedish term *lagom* means "not too little, not too much," a concept that is particularly useful when we're changing our habits.

Doing anything new is hard for most people, and biting off more than we can chew just makes it harder—if not impossible. In fact, it can be so overwhelming that we don't even try. On the other hand, if you take small, manageable steps, you will be moving forward with joy. You don't always have to be amazing; just start small and enjoy the ride.

For example: let's say you aspire to become a writer. You can't expect to write a book immediately. You have to sit and write something (almost) every day for as long as it will take you. I used that thinking as I was writing this book. Do what you can to move in the right direction and feel good about what you've done. Or, if you aspire to cut out sweets but you love cake and ice cream, start by cutting back rather than eliminating them from your diet entirely. Anything forbidden automatically becomes that much more desirable, so the thing to do is to reduce—maybe start by having a piece of cake or a scoop of ice cream every other day, then maybe every third day, or only on Saturdays.

There are always small things you can do that produce immediate changes for the better.

PLAN TO FAIL

No one's perfect. There will always be bumps in the road, detours, plans that go awry. So, you need to prepare to fail from time to time and you need a contingency plan for getting yourself back on track. For example, I like to run 20 minutes twice a week, and when I don't feel like it, I tell myself that it is OK to walk. Maybe that's just me, but it's still a good example of how I personally get out there—running or walking is not the point. What matters is that I don't get completely out of the habit I'm trying to make an important part of my lifestyle.

THE FOUR PILLARS OF OVERALL HEALTH

Although the particulars will certainly vary from one person to the next, I believe there are four areas in everyone's life where making small changes will create big results. These are what I call the four pillars of overall health—eating, sleeping, breathing, and moving—and, in the chapters that follow, I'll be discussing their functions and how you can fortify them by changing your habits one small step at a time.

SUMMARY OF CHAPTER 3

1   Habits are actions we perform automatically without much conscious thought.

2   Awareness is crucial for change: it's important to recognize what it is you actually want to do in order to develop new habits that will lead to transformation.

3   Create new habits step by step. When creating new habits, start small and take manageable steps.

4   Understand the gap between where you are now and where you want to be, and look for opportunities to succeed.

5   Make an effort to surround yourself with individuals that share your aspirations and desired way of life.

PART 2

FOUR PILLARS TO SUPPORT OVERALL HEALTH

THE 4 PILLARS

1 EAT

[*äta*]

Page 62

2 SLEEP

[*sömn*]

Page 98

3

BREATHE

[*andas*]

Page 114

4

MOVE

[*rörelse*]

Page 130

CHAPTER

4

HOW, WHEN, WHAT TO EAT

EAT

[*äta*]

don't want you to think that any one of my four pillars of holistic health is more important than the others, but I'm starting out with eating because it seems to me that, of the four, this is the one causing most of our health problems today. And, as I've said, your mouth is the gateway to your entire body; everything that goes into your body starts in your mouth.

According to the CDC, chronic diseases account for about 90 percent of healthcare spending in the United States. Most of our chronic diseases can be reversed, reduced, or eliminated by lifestyle modifications in general and eating in particular. Almost all of us would do well to examine how and what we eat, and to find ways to improve our relationship with food. It truly is that important.

With all of this in mind, I will be sharing with you suggestions on what foods to eat to promote your oral health and, therefore, your overall health. I hope you find my practical ideas useful when you are implementing new habits for your aspired lifestyle. That said, this is *not*, I want to emphasize, a diet book. In fact, the word "diet" has such a negative connotation that I hesitate to use it at all. Food is, and should be, a source of not only physical health but also social and emotional nourishment, and should not be associated with deprivation.

WHY DO YOU EAT?

Changing your habits related to food and eating—like changing any habit—requires intentionality. You need to think about why you do something in a particular way in order to come up with another way of doing it that will, with time, become equally habitual and even more rewarding.

Food serves us in many ways. It literally nourishes every cell in the body. It is the clock by which we set the rhythm of our days: time for breakfast, time for lunch, time for dinner. And it brings us together not only with family and friends but also as a culture. It is at the center of almost every kind of gathering, from a business lunch to a holiday feast. Eating is also one of the few things we do that has the ability to engage, activate, and stimulate all of our five senses: smell, touch, taste, sight, and hearing, which is yet another reason for my obsession with the mouth area as the gateway to life.

"

A memorable gathering is more than the proper table setting, menu, and décor. The magic lies in the connection created between people.

—Priya Parker, author of *The Art of Gathering*

Given how ubiquitous and essential food is in your life, it will be helpful to ask yourself a few questions about your eating habits:

- How can I make the act of eating more nutritious?

- How can I make more time to find the joy in cooking and sharing a meal with loved ones?

- How can I make my meals less functional and more fun?

I can already hear you saying: but where will I find the time? I'd argue that ultimately with this approach you can save time; you just have to be thoughtful and to make a plan. My approach to how I feed myself and my family is relatively simple. By taking ten minutes at the start of my week to make a plan and a grocery list, I head into my week feeling confident and prepared. And as with my other advice, I invite you to take it and make it your own. Use it as a starting point for the new you.

Each meal isn't a chore, but an opportunity. We have multiple opportunities every day: breakfast, lunch, and dinner. This happens every day, every week, every month, and every year. Your decisions around your meals, therefore, add up! Making small changes to your habits can create powerful momentum.

If you create a solid routine, it becomes second nature. No more opening the fridge and not knowing what to make. You can make things easy for yourself. If you give yourself some guidelines with the intention to feed your body more nutritious food as easily as possible, it will make a difference over time.

Feeding yourself and your loved ones doesn't need to be stressful. Find a few go-to, wholesome meals that you feel comfortable making. I share some of my favorite recipes with you on page 146.

FOOD AS MEDICINE

"Let food be thy medicine and medicine be thy food," is a quote most often attributed to the ancient Greek physician Hippocrates. Initially, thinking of food as medicine may not sound very appealing. Taking medicine is something we do because we have to. Eating is something we think of as pleasurable (unless, of course, it's the spinach your mother made you finish before you could have dessert). But what if the food you enjoy eating could also prevent you from having to take that medicine? The fact is that, in many cases, it can—and does. Early in the 21st century, science has become clear on this issue: not only how much but also what you eat can reduce your chances of getting any number of chronic diseases, including diabetes, cardiovascular disease, and some cancers, to name just a few.

I don't know how other families operate, but we gathered our children—who were between the ages of 8 and 12 at the time—and discussed the "Family Rules" that ought to be posted in our house. We came up with these guidelines after deliberating and casting our votes, in order to serve as a reminder of what we believe to be vital for our family.

OUR FAMILY RULES
(created with our kids)

1. Love each other.
2. Move your body.
3. Study and practise.
4. Life is for giving.
5. Response-ability.

The rules changed when our children were all grown up and as we "evolved." Today the family rules we have in our house are as follows:

OUR CURRENT FAMILY RULES

1. You are what you eat eats.
2. You are who you are with.
3. You are what you believe.

> *It seems clear to me that more and more people are finding value in exploring ways to eat and live better. Unfortunately, we still have a lot to unpack.*

As a culture, particularly in the West, our lives have been saturated (literally) with processed foods, sugary foods, and too much food that tastes good while we're eating it but may make us feel bad, or even sick, in the longer term.

It was fascinating for me to learn that Dr Weston Price, a *dentist* in Cleveland, Ohio, uncovered the link between food and medicine as far back as the 1930s—long before the current "food as medicine" movement. By observing the eating habits of isolated communities in 14 different countries around the world, Price found that so long as they stuck to their traditional diets, which were universally and naturally rich in essential nutrients, these indigenous peoples typically had straight teeth, free from decay, and overall good health. But once they began moving to more "civilized" towns and cities and adopting more "modernized" (read: processed) diets—consisting mainly of white flour products, sugar, white rice, jams, canned goods, and vegetable fats—they also began producing children who had lost the oral and overall good health enjoyed by previous generations.

Similar findings have been more recently published by National Geographic Fellow Dan Buettner, who identified what he has called "Blue Zones"—the five places in the world where people live longest—and made a study of their lifestyle habits. What he found is that certain habits are common in all of these zones, and he posits that these can add ten years to your life. He called these habits "the Blue Zone Power of 9."

The bases for his findings have been called into question, but, whether following his rules is going to cause you to become a centenarian, there is certainly enough good, logical information here to be of benefit to almost anyone. Only one of Buettner's recommendations is specifically food-related, as you can see on the next page in my interpretation of these rules.

THE BLUE ZONE POWER OF 9

Buettner's Rules (As I Define Them)

1 MOVE NATURALLY

Make physical activity like walking or gardening a part of your daily routine that you don't have to think about. There's no need for intensive workouts.

___

2 PURPOSE

Have a purpose in life. Doing so makes you happier, healthier, and helps you live longer.

___

3 DOWNSHIFT

Build stress-relieving rituals into your routine so that your body can recover physically. (See *Fika* on page 72)

___

4 80 PERCENT RULE

Stop eating when you're 80 percent full. The 20 percent difference can determine whether you gain or lose weight.

___

5 PLANT SLANT

Eat more beans, vegetables, fruits, and whole grains. Meat should be consumed in small amounts.

6 WINE

Drink some red wine in moderation on some or most days. *Lagom* is what seems to work here for those of us who feel OK about drinking alcohol.

——

7 BELONG

Be part of a community to improve your well-being and life expectancy.

——

8 LOVED ONES FIRST

Make family a priority, and invest in them with love and care.

——

9 RIGHT TRIBE

Be surrounded by close friends and people who share and/or support your healthy lifestyle habits.

The point is that eating or living better is not rocket science. Our human biology has not changed much since the time of the ancient Greeks (and probably longer), but our lifestyle has changed very rapidly in just the last 50 years, and not in a healthy way.

FIKA

No, that's not a typo. It's a Swedish tradition that translates to "coffee break" but is really much more than that. It's a concept, some would even say a ritual, that is an important part of Swedish culture. It is the intentional act of taking a pause and enjoying life. It's an opportunity to slow down, connect, and catch up with friends or peers at work. When I worked as a dentist in Stockholm, one of my favorite parts of the workday was taking a scheduled *fika* to gather with my coworkers in the designated "fika room" at the clinic, for a cup of tea or coffee.

Many Swedes actually consider it almost essential to make time for *fika* every day. And to be clear, if you have your coffee alone at your desk, that is not *fika*, it's just coffee. In fact, what you're consuming is less important than the fact that you're taking the time to connect and socialize with others. *Fika* is often accompanied by some type of food, such as a *bulle* (cinnamon roll) or perhaps a chocolate ball. The only caveat is that whatever it is, it should be fresh, not too much, nicely presented, and preferably homemade. Again, the emphasis is on the enjoyment of the moment, as much as the pleasure of the food itself.

Make it a habit to eat off a real plate, with a placemat, and why not a cloth napkin, whenever you can. My grandfather taught me to make the effort out of respect for the food, and to take a moment of "self care."

For me as an example... Ever since we got married, my husband and I have tried our best to make Friday night dinners special for our family and friends. But special doesn't have to mean complicated; it just needs to be thoughtful. In fact, we typically serve the same food each week: chicken soup, roasted chicken and vegetables, and a chewy chocolate brownie with berries and whipped cream—a dessert I've been making since the 1980s. We started making the same dinner because of convenience and lack of time. Now, because of all the memories we have of eating it together, it has come to occupy a special place in our hearts. Even my grown children ask for the same foods when they come to visit. Love that! How have we made this happen over the years? We prep most of the food a night or two before, and whenever we can we make sure to make enough to freeze for the next week.

In order to be truly nourishing, eating should be intentional. It's too bad, for both our physical and emotional health, that in these hectic modern times, when so many of us spend most of our lives multitasking, eating is often something we do while we're doing something else. For many, that means eating at their desk while working, or in the car while driving (which isn't a very good idea for many reasons). But even if it's while we're sitting in front of the television, which we think is relaxing, it means we're still multi-processing and not giving our full attention to either the food or the TV.

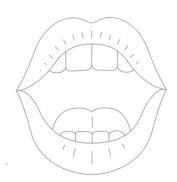

WHEN DO YOU EAT?

I know there are many reasons why you can't choose when you eat every meal every day. But I'm going to give you some guidelines for making the best choices whenever you are able to choose.

My best advice is to eat two or three "real" or main meals per day—such as breakfast, lunch, and dinner. You may want a small meal in addition, if you find one is needed somewhere in between. You probably call that "snacks." (More about that in a minute.)

You've probably heard of intermittent fasting, which has become popular these days. I typically do not want to label the way I'm eating. But in fact, intermittent fasting at a basic level is just making sure to have a long stretch between your last meal of the day and your first meal the next day. This seems like simple good sense and is what I would recommend as a dentist anyway (no matter what you call it) to any of my clients, since it is a very good idea for your oral health. As we've already discussed, saliva is the primary oral cleanser, and it needs time between meals to restore the proper pH balance in your mouth and also remineralize your teeth by providing essential minerals, such as calcium and phosphate, in order to prevent cavities. As we produce less saliva at night, while we're sleeping, it is important, not only to help you get to sleep but also to maintain oral health, that you not eat anything for a couple of hours before bedtime.

For all of these reasons, I would suggest that if you have no medical restrictions, you try intermittent fasting at a *lagom* (or moderate) level. Here's what I recommend:

Your first meal of the day should be at least 12 to 14 hours after you finish your dinner the day before. For example, you might eat dinner between 6 and 7 p.m. and then have breakfast the next day between 7 and 8 a.m. In between, you can drink water, or black coffee or tea without any sugar.

Ideally, eat only at mealtimes. If you feel the need, you could have one extra small meal a day. Although I personally find that when I eat breakfast later—say at 10 a.m.—I don't feel the need to eat as frequently for the rest of the day.

So, your day could look something like this (assuming your bedtime is around 10 to 11 p.m.):

7:30 to 9 a.m.	Coffee / tea
9 to 10 a.m.	Breakfast
1 to 2 p.m.	Lunch
6 to 7 p.m.	Dinner
10 to 11 p.m.	Bedtime

Always start your day with a glass of room-temperature water. Drinking water in the morning can help to improve hydration, boost metabolism, enhance cognitive function, support digestion, and promote detoxification.

And there you have it! The *lagom* approach to intermittent fasting. Nothing too extreme, but it allows enough time overnight for your mouth to "reset" in order to maintain oral health.

THE TROUBLE WITH SNACKING

Americans snack a lot. When my family moved here, I was surprised to learn that it was a parental duty to take snacks to our children's sporting events. I didn't really want to celebrate their achievements with a doughnut, so I said that if I had to contribute, I would bring something healthy like an apple. My kids, of course, were mortified. Oh well.

The trouble with snacking is at least in part related to the word itself. "Snack" or "snacking" allows us to pretend that what's going in our mouth isn't really food. And very often, at least in terms of nutritional value, it really *isn't* food. I know that there's been a lot of talk lately about "healthy snacks," but I'd still prefer to call them small meals.

There are two main problems with these small meals. First is the quality of the snacks themselves. Snacks tend to be portable, packaged, and shelf-stable. This often means that they are filled with processed, unhealthy ingredients, and wrapped in packaging that is damaging to our environment. Second, most typical snacks include refined sugar and other highly processed carbohydrates, which cause a quick spike in blood sugar levels, followed by a steep drop, causing us to become hungrier sooner than if we ate something that took longer to digest. There are many good studies indicating that eating snacks, or at least the foods most people eat as snacks, is not helpful to our overall health.

HOW DO YOU EAT?

When we think about the benefits of eating, we often think about nutrition. But when it comes to oral and overall health, there's more to the picture than meets the eye. And as a dentist, "how" you eat can take a different and more literal meaning. Chewing your food (also known as mastication) is essential for good oral health and optimal overall health.

DIGESTION

Chewing is the first step in the digestion process. It breaks down food into smaller particles, increasing the surface area for enzymes to act upon. The mechanical action of chewing mixes food with saliva. Properly chewed food is easier for the digestive system to process, enhancing nutrient absorption and overall digestion.

NUTRIENT EXTRACTION

Chewing food thoroughly helps release nutrients from the food you are eating, making them more available to the body for absorption. Chewing aids in the release of vital nutrients, vitamins, and minerals found in food.

ORAL HEALTH

Chewing promotes good oral health by stimulating saliva production. Saliva helps to neutralize acids, wash away food particles, and prevent tooth decay. It also contains antimicrobial components that help control oral bacteria.

CHEWING HELPS YOU EAT THE RIGHT AMOUNT OF FOOD

When chewing, you are sending signals to the brain, triggering a sense of fullness and satisfaction. Chewing also allows you to savor the taste of food, promoting mindful eating and preventing overeating.

JAW HEALTH AND STRENGTH

Regular chewing exercises the jaw muscles, promoting their strength and maintaining proper alignment of the jaw. This can contribute to improved jaw function, reduced jaw pain, and a decreased risk of temporomandibular joint (TMJ) disorders.

Overall, chewing is essential for efficient digestion, nutrient absorption, oral health, appetite regulation, and jaw strength. Incorporating mindful chewing habits and consuming a variety of chewable foods can positively impact overall health and well-being.

66

The mechanical forces generated by chewing food not only help your jaws grow to the right size and shape, they also help your teeth fit properly within the jaw. Changes in chewing changed human jaws and faces.

—Daniel Lieberman

99

The types of food we eat make a difference to the way we chew. And as we grow and develop, the way and frequency with which we chew helps to shape our facial structures. Our bone development is dependent on chewing, which engages our facial muscles. This, in turn, gives us the shape and space in the jaw for our teeth.

WHAT DO YOU EAT?

Aha, I can hear you thinking, now she's going to hit us with the tough stuff. But, as I've said, this is not a diet book, and I have no intention of dictating what you should be eating at every meal. My goal here is to share practical solutions and suggestions with a focus on what is good for your optimal oral health, and, therefore, also your overall health.

There are a lot of fads, trends, and ideas related to what to eat, most of which are confusing to the point of exhaustion. And not very helpful. From not eating fat to eating more fat. From eating more bread (as was advertised by the government health organization in Sweden when I was younger) to eating less bread. From eating no meat to eating more meat (for health reasons, not animal welfare, I might add). From eating no eggs to eating plenty of eggs. No wonder we are all a bit lost.

Of course, scientific progress is not always linear, and new data informs new advice. However, what is the end result for all of us trying to live better and live well? Utter confusion!

Some of the most helpful and actionable advice around food I have found is from Michael Pollan (author, journalist, and professor of the Practice of Non-Fiction and journalism at prestigious schools in America), who has also written some wonderful books about our relationship with food. In one of them, *In Defense of Food*, he summarized what we ought to eat in seven words that I believe say it all.

> ## Eat food. Not too much. Mostly plants.
>
> **—Michael Pollan**

These words became wildly quoted and used, and the popularity inspired Michael to write *Food Rules: An Eater's Manual*. In this later book he expanded on the seven words to include 64 rules. Below I have listed a few of my favorites, which act as inspiration for how I think about eating and living well.

PART 1: WHAT SHOULD I EAT?
- Don't eat anything your great-grandmother wouldn't recognize as food.
- If it came from a plant, eat it; if it was made in a plant, don't.

PART 2: WHAT KIND OF FOOD SHOULD I EAT?
- Sweeten and salt your food yourself.
- Eat all the junk food you want, as long as you cook it yourself.

PART 3: HOW SHOULD I EAT?
- Eat less.
- Eat meals.

"Break the rules once in a while" (my favorite!)

I love these rules and have found myself able to incorporate them into my life easily, and to great benefit. Based on these, I've developed some additional guidelines that I also now live by:

- Chew your food properly.
- Don't eat on the go!
- Don't snack; eat meals.
- Don't eat too close to bedtime.
- Make your food beautiful.
- Eat together with others.

I believe the best way to eat healthier overall is to eat more home-cooked meals. While we all enjoy going to restaurants, it is also true that when we eat outside the home, we have less control over what ingredients are in the food. An additional benefit of home cooking is that we often consume those meals with the people we love most. And if we live alone, it's a great excuse to invite them to join us. People enjoy going to other people's homes and being treated to a meal. The food doesn't have to be fancy or time-consuming to prepare. In fact, I believe that the best meals are those based on a variety of simply cooked vegetables, which provide lots of color as well as lots of flavor, with some meat, chicken, or fish (or whatever your personal preference is).

To make this a reality, you could start a cooking group in which each of you cooks one day of the week for the group. There are several great ways of doing this to make it happen in a joyful and practical way.

SUGAR OR FAT: AN ONGOING DEBATE

For many years, our relationship with sugar and fat has been, well, let us just say *complicated*. Maybe you grew up with your mother telling you that candy was going to rot your teeth. Or perhaps you've been trying to stick to a low-fat diet because you think that eating fat makes you fat.

The fact is that all carbohydrates, from vegetables to table sugar, are metabolized as glucose—in other words, sugar. When your body senses glucose in your bloodstream, it signals to your pancreas to produce insulin, which, in turn, moves the glucose out of your blood and into your cells to use as energy. Problems start when you produce more glucose than you need for energy

In Sweden, we have a tradition that kids enjoy their sweet treats on Saturdays. We call it *lördags godis* (Saturday candy). For most younger children, it is the only day when they eat candy in the week. Don't take it too literally though; there is room for dessert occasionally after dinner, and the Swedish version of "snacks" in the afternoon for children as well. The "snacks" I talked about earlier in this chapter are looked upon as small meals rather than sweet treats.

As a dentist and a parent, I thought it was a great idea to stick to *lördags godis* for my kids when they were little. My logic was that candy is most commonly consumed between meals, which would expose the children to sugar more frequently, which would cause a pH drop and therefore a higher risk of cavities.

(maybe because you ate the whole birthday cake instead of just a slice). When that happens, your body still keeps producing insulin, which is also a fat-storage hormone. So, bottom line: too much glucose leads to too much insulin leads to too much fat!

In the end, eating either too much sugar or too much fat will make you fat. But eating too much of either fat or sugar can also make you sick, increasing your risk for heart disease and/or diabetes, to name just a couple. However, both fat and sugar add flavor to food. So, typically, when processed-food producers cut out fat, they add more sugar, which is the problem with so many low-fat foods.

The ingredients that become popular in the foods we eat are influenced by social conditions. Decision-makers, lobbyists, and manufacturing powers have huge sway in the American (and Western) diet overall. As packaged and processed foods gained popularity in the 1950s, a scientific debate between sugar-rich and fat-rich foods was center stage. But why did fat become the villain for so long?

Let's take a closer look and, hopefully, arrive at a more balanced and, therefore, more helpful approach to the problem.

In the 1960s and 1970s, epidemiologist Dr. Ancel Keys and physiologist, nutritionist, and physician Dr. John Yudkin were trying to determine the reason for the increase in cardiovascular disease and weight gain. In America, Dr. Keys was focusing on high cholesterol and saturated fat as the underlying reasons for increasing weight gain; while, in England, Dr. Yudkin was looking at excessive consumption of sugar as the main problem. Both Yudkin and his book *Pure, White and Deadly* came under a barrage of criticism from the sugar industry, the manufacturers of processed foods, and from Ancel Keys.

Over the years, as the "fat theory" gained acceptance in the food industry, causing the creation of an entire low-fat movement within an industry, as virtually all foods were stripped of their fat content. But there were two nasty, unintended consequences of this shift. First, fat is a carrier of taste by helping to dissolve and concentrate flavor. So, in order to make foods, for example yogurt, taste good, sugar was added to everything from which the fat had been removed. The second problem was that fat increases satiety. It makes us feel full, so the net effect was that good-tasting food made us feel less full, leading to the creation of larger and larger portions.

Fortunately, more and more scientists are now revisiting their earlier conclusions, and it is becoming clear that consuming "good" fats and less sugar/carbs will disrupt the epidemic of obesity plaguing so many of our current societies. As with anything else, *lagom* is the answer. Neither too much sugar nor too much fat is good for us. I think most people know that to be true.

Drawing on my own experience and understanding, I would say that there are four key areas where adjustments are helpful:

Fewer processed carbohydrates: Be aware of what carbohydrates you are eating. Try to decrease the intake of carbohydrates in general, especially those coming from highly processed foods.

Less sugar intake: Look for sugar everywhere, not only in the obvious places such as cakes, cookies, chocolates (my favorite!), etc., but oftentimes in unexpected places. There is added sugar in almost all packaged foods, as well as in peanut butter, ketchup, and many more staples most of us have at home.

I am separating sugars and carbs for simplicity and practical reasons, but, as many of you know, sugar is a form of carbohydrate.

More vegetables: We just don't eat enough of them. They are our biggest health promoters, and we can eat as many of the non-starchy vegetables as we want. Eat a rainbow of colored vegetables! Eat them raw, steamed, or grilled. Make them your main course. Meat and fish should be side dishes, not the other way around.

Better fats: We have been fooled into believing that fats are what make you fat. But that isn't always true. You don't become green from eating greens and you don't become fat from eating fat. Eating the right kinds of fat is important for satiety and for managing hunger and energy. Olive oil, nut butters, avocado, and grass-fed butter are great forms of fat when consumed in the right amounts. I am not a fan of the processed vegetable oils that are so common in most foods because these vegetable oils are high in omega-6 fatty acids, which the body needs, but unfortunately, when you have too much omega-6, particularly when the omega-6 to omega-3 fatty acid ratio is uneven, it might increase inflammation in the body.* Another consideration is that when vegetable oils are processed, they can be exposed to high heat, light, and oxygen, resulting in oxidation and the formation of hazardous chemicals such as free radicals. Oxidated oils can cause inflammation and oxidative stress in the body, which have been linked to a variety of chronic disorders.

Note that not all vegetable oils are equally unhealthy. Certain oils, such as extra-virgin olive oil and coconut oil, are considered healthier options due to their lower omega-6 content and higher stability. Try to find these oils and minimize the consumption of highly processed vegetable oils that can be found in a lot of dressings.

---

* Meat is omega-3 when the animal eats grass, but omega-6 when the animal eats corn. Fish is omega-3; chicken is omega-6. The first new fatty acid chain discovery in 70 years is something called C15 (also known as 'fatty 15'). It's three times more potent than omega-3 and something I now take daily. For full disclosure, we like this so much that our family is a small investor in the company.

SOME SURPRISING FACTS ABOUT SUGAR

Sugar in and of itself does not cause cavities. What does have a detrimental effect on your teeth and gums are the acids produced by the bacteria that break down the carbs and sugar you eat. So once again, it's an issue of your saliva being able to reset the pH balance in your mouth. Your job is to avoid eating sugar too often or too much, to give your saliva a fighting chance against the bacteria.

> *And here's another newsflash:*
> *All sugars—even naturally occurring sugars—cause problems when consumed in large quantities and not in their natural form.*

So, for example, you may have heard the saying "An apple a day keeps the doctor away." Note that it does not say "Drink four ounces of apple juice a day." This is because consuming fruit as juice means that you are consuming the juice of several apples, without the fiber that slows down digestion so that your blood sugar doesn't spike and so that you feel fuller for longer. The same holds true for other whole fruits and their juices.

Or think about dried fruit. As a dentist, one reason I'm not in favor of dried fruits is that they stick to your teeth and feed the bacteria involved in giving you cavities and gum disease. But on top of that, we seem to think that because they're fruits, they must be healthy, and so we tend to consume too many. But, of course, the sugar in fruit is still sugar, and when the fruit is dried, that sugar becomes more concentrated. So, just as it's better to eat an apple than it is to drink apple juice, it's better to eat a fresh apricot (or any other fruit) than to eat a handful of dried ones.

SUGARS GO BY MANY NAMES

- Agave nectar
- Glucose solids
- Barbados sugar
- Golden sugar
- Barley malt
- Golden syrup
- Barley malt syrup
- Grape sugar
- Beet sugar
- High-fructose corn syrup (HFCS)
- Brown sugar
- Icing sugar
- Buttered syrup
- Cane juice
- Malt syrup
- Castor sugar
- Maltodextrin
- Coconut palm sugar
- Maltol
- Coconut sugar
- Molasses
- Confectioner's sugar
- Muscovado
- Corn sweetener
- Palm sugar
- Corn syrup
- Refiner's syrup
- Date sugar
- Rice syrup
- Dextrin
- Saccharose
- Dextrose
- Sorghum syrup
- Evaporated cane juice
- Sweet sorghum
- Free-flowing brown sugars
- Syrup
- Fructose
- Treacle
- Fruit juice concentrate
- Turbinado sugar
- Yellow sugar

NOW, WHAT ABOUT FAT?

Well, first of all, you may have been told that fat makes you fat and should be avoided at all costs. Fortunately, as I mentioned earlier, we are coming to terms with the fact that this is not the whole truth. We need dietary fats for energy, to keep us warm, to support the integrity of our cells, and for our brain health. Fat also serves to protect our vital organs and helps our body absorb other nutrients, including the fat-soluble vitamins A, D, E, and K.

Besides the health benefits from fats, they also make you feel satiated throughout the day.

Eating a *lagom* amount of the fats that benefit our oral and overall health is what we aim for.

Diving into what fats to eat for good health over the past 15 years, I have tried hard not to go with the next trend or fad, but to listen to those thought leaders I really trust and do my own research. One of my sources regarding what to eat and what not to eat has been Dr. Mark Hyman, whose important recommendations about which fats to focus on in cooking, and which to limit or avoid, have become words that I live by.

FATS TO EAT:

- Organic extra-virgin olive oil
- Organic avocado oil
- Walnut oil
- Almond oil
- Macadamia oil
- Unrefined sesame oil
- Tahini (sesame seed paste)
- Flax oil
- Hemp oil
- Avocado, olives, and other plant sources of fat
- Nuts and seeds
- Butter from pastured, grass-fed cows and goats
- Grass-fed ghee
- Organic, humanely raised tallow, lard, duck fat or chicken fat.
- Coconut oil or MCT (medium chain triglycerides) oil
- Sustainable palm oil (look for certified sustainable palm oil)

FATS TO AVOID OR LIMIT:

- Soybean oil
- Canola oil
- Corn oil
- Safflower oil
- Sunflower oil
- Peanut oil
- Vegetable oil, grapeseed oil
- Margarine, and butter substitutes
- Anything that says "hydrogenated"

From *The Pegan Diet* by Mark Hyman

WHAT DOES PROTEIN DO FOR YOU?

Proteins are important for more than just maintaining healthy muscles and bones. They also make us feel full after eating; your level of the hunger hormone ghrelin is decreased by protein. In addition to this, proteins have a role to play in maintaining good oral health. Protein-rich foods provide calcium phosphate, vitamin K2, vitamin D3, and vitamin A, each of which is beneficial to your oral health. We tend to think of meat when we think of protein, but fish as well as many plants also provide a powerful punch of protein, if you're able to eat a combination of grains, legumes, seeds, nuts, and vegetables. And it's easy to make a simple change, like substituting a breakfast high in carbohydrates with food that is high in protein instead, such as egg, or Greek yogurt with nuts and seeds.

Here are some protein-based strategies I use to eat protein mindfully:

- When I look to consume meat, I try to eat a variety of grass-fed meats, including wild meats like deer and elk, which can often be found in the frozen food department.

- I look for fish and seafood from safe and sustainable sources.

- I buy poultry and eggs that are from regenerative farms and/or pasture-raised.

- I try to source dairy as much as I can from A2 cow milk, sheep and/or grass-fed cow milk.

- I have been adding protein to my first meal shake lately to boost my protein intake.

TAKE YOUR VITAMINS
(in food, and supplements if needed)

For the longest time I thought I could eat what I needed to stay healthy. Since I started having grandchildren, I caved in and have been taking some basic vitamins, such as vitamin D and magnesium, to keep me as fit and healthy as possible in order to keep up with my grandchildren.

In his book *The Dental Diet*, Dr. Steven Lin states that "the foods that are good for your teeth are good for your whole body." And that would certainly include foods that contribute to the healthy development of your facial bones: the frontal bone, the nose bone, the cheekbone, the upper jawbone, and the lower jawbone. Those would be foods that contain vitamins A, D, C, and K2, as well as the mineral calcium.

VITAMIN A

In addition to helping the membranes of your skin, eyes, mouth, nose, and lungs remain moist, vitamin A contributes to the development of your teeth and bones. It can be found in fish, egg yolks, and liver, as well as leafy green vegetables and oranges, or other orange-colored foods which contain high levels of beta-carotene that your body converts into vitamin A.

VITAMIN D

As well as helping you to absorb calcium and thus boost bone mineral density in the mouth, vitamin D in conjunction with calcium helps protect and contribute to healthy gum tissue and assists in preventing dental caries (cavities) by carrying the calcium into the enamel when needed.

Vitamin D also helps to protect older adults from developing osteoporosis, and strengthens the body against respiratory infections, cancer, heart disease, diabetes, and other illnesses.

When exposed to sunshine, your body produces vitamin D, but you can also acquire it by eating fatty fish, canned tuna, herring (a Swedish favorite), egg yolks, portobello mushrooms.

VITAMIN C

Although it's commonly known for helping to fight the common cold, vitamin C is essential for the maintenance and repair of your bones, teeth, and especially your gums. Aside from citrus fruits, which I'm sure you already know about, you can also get vitamin C from potatoes and leafy greens.

VITAMIN K2

Vitamin K2 was discovered in 1929 and first described in a German scientific magazine under the term *Koagulations vitamin*, which gave rise to the name vitamin K. Furthermore, while researching indigenous diets, Dr. Weston Price discovered that this "new vitamin-like activator" (now known as vitamin K2) provided protection against tooth decay. We now know that this happens because K2 assists in the deposition of calcium in the teeth. K2 is also involved in calcium metabolism regulation in the body. It aids in directing calcium to the bones and teeth rather than collecting it in soft tissues. Food sources of vitamin K2 include dairy products, animal products, and fermented foods.

To summarize, vitamin K2 is now commonly associated with calcium metabolism, bone health, and cardiovascular health. Vitamin K, and particularly K2, is essential for blood coagulation.

"The fundamental role of vitamin K2 in the skeletal system means it should be at the center of a strategy to prevent crooked teeth in future generations."

—Dr. Steven Lin

CALCIUM (AND PHOSPHATE)

This is important for remineralizing and hardening tooth enamel and strengthening your jawbone. The only caveat is that if your mouth becomes too acidic because you are constantly drinking or snacking, it will keep calling out for calcium, which could cause an excess of calcium in your bloodstream, potentially leading to weaker bones, kidney stones, and heart problems.

Milk, cheese, and yogurt, as well as broccoli, carrots, and salmon are all good sources of calcium.

ARE YOU READY TO MAKE NEW HABITS?

EAT YOUR VEGETABLES

We can probably all agree that including more plant foods in your regular diet is a definite way to enhance your dental and general health. Look for alkaline foods, such as arugula and cucumber, that have a higher pH level, meaning they are less acidic and more basic. They will not only include a range of vitamins and minerals that your teeth and gums, as well as your stomach, require to thrive, but also help you keep your pH stable in your mouth.

TAKE AWAY TEMPTATION

Go through your kitchen and remove the foods that are tempting you to eat them when you know you really shouldn't—such as cookies, candy, sauces, fried foods, and others that are full of refined sugar or are highly processed.

BECOME A SAVVY SHOPPER

It's important to read the label on anything that comes in a package, and make it your business to know what it all means.

See, for example, the many names for refined sugar listed on page 87. Another trick is to not be hungry when you are grocery shopping. There are also some great apps to help you find recipes and make sharable grocery lists, such as Epicurious and Whisk.

WHOLE FOODS ARE HEALTHY FOR YOU AND THE PLANET

Whole foods are those food items that arrive in the store looking pretty much the way they grew. Very often they're displayed on the shelves without any packaging, which means less plastic will be added to the planet when you dispose of your trash.

PLAN AHEAD

This may be the most important tip I can give you. It's when you don't have anything in the house to eat that you're most likely to pick up some food for dinner or stop at the deli for a doughnut on the way to work. If you can come up with a shopping list and a week's worth of menus, you can shop once a week, prepare things in advance, and, therefore, be much more likely to stick with your plan.

REDUCE SUGAR INTAKE

Whatever you eat, try to figure out if it has any hidden sugar. It can be sugar by some other name (see page 87) and it can be added to something you never thought would have sugar in it. Examples are bread, dressings, sauces, and anything ready-made, to name a few.

AVOID THE UNHEALTHY FATS

Look out for the processed vegetable oils mentioned earlier that you want to eat as little of as possible. Start reading the labels on all food items you consider buying. Don't forget to check all the premade food, boxed or not, before you consider bringing it home.

SUMMARY OF CHAPTER 4

1   Michael Pollan's advice around food has had a huge impact on my way of thinking about food. "Eat food. Not too much. Mostly plants."

2   pH levels: When you eat or drink, especially foods high in sugars or carbohydrates, the bacteria in your mouth can produce acids as they break down these substances. This leads to a temporary decrease in pH levels, making the mouth more acidic. The acidity creates an environment where harmful bacteria can thrive, increasing the risk of dental issues like tooth decay and gum disease.

3   Snacking: Try not to snack throughout the day but instead eat bigger meals.

4   Chewing your food: Properly chewed food is easier for the digestive system to process, enhancing nutrient absorption and overall digestion. Chewing stimulates your saliva, which promotes your oral health as it washes away food particles and provides the mouth with antimicrobial components.

EAT: HABITS WORKSHEET

CONNECT

Write down your top 3 aspirations for your life

Example: I want to improve my overall health

_____

_____

_____

_____

_____

CURATE

What habits do you want to practice? List a few habits that you would consider trying as a way to reach your aspirations. Remember to identify habits that are small, doable, and practical (realistic). Also favor habits that can be integrated into your existing daily routines.

Examples: Eat vegetables everyday. Eat chocolate only on Saturdays.

_____

_____

_____

_____

_____

_____

_____

CREATE

Now, when you are set on what new habits you want to commit to, consider the context of your life and make sure you remove all reasons to say no and make it as easy as you can to say yes!

Example: I commit to include vegetables in every meal I eat by having vegetables available in my fridge.

What? _____

_____

When? _____

How? _____

_____

I commit to: _____

_____

_____

_____

_____

_____

_____

_____

CELEBRATE

Be your own cheerleader! Every day you practice the habit, you will celebrate with a pat on the shoulder and say "Well done!"

THE TRUTH ABOUT SLEEP

SLEEP

[*sömn*]

I n the words of Matthew Walker, neuroscientist and author of *Why We Sleep*, "Sleep is one of the most important but least understood aspects of our life, wellness, and longevity." If you think about it, the relationship between your oral health and the quality of your sleep ought to be fairly obvious. After all, one of the most common and universal aspects of a pre-sleep routine is brushing your teeth before bed. The same goes for when you wake up. Brushing your teeth is key to your feeling refreshed and prepared for the day. This is no coincidence! The way we sleep affects the way we breathe, the breath itself, our oral microbiome, and our tongue posture—in other words, our oral health. And of course, the reverse is also true, in that our oral health can impact the quality of our sleep. And by improving our sleep, we're also improving our overall health.

Yet we are living in the middle of a sleep-deprivation epidemic.

"Over one-third of adults do not get a sufficient amount of sleep. Insufficient sleep has been linked to a number of chronic conditions including type 2 diabetes, hypertension, coronary heart disease, stroke, obesity, and depression. Luckily there are a number of habits that can help you get a good night's sleep"

—Wayne Giles, Dean of the School of Public Health, UIC

And yet while some people bemoan the fact that they have trouble sleeping, others seem to be equally happy to not sleep at all. They seem to wear sleep deprivation as a kind of badge of honor. But, despite the fact that I know how important it is to get a good night's sleep, I understand where they're coming from. We all live hectic lives, trying to fit in time for work, family, friends, and, these days, increasing screen time. So, I get it. But you can't multitask while you're sleeping. Despite all the advances in technology, no one's figured that out yet.

Have you ever had the experience of putting on a pair of glasses for the first time and being amazed to see what you've been missing? The same may be true of sleep. If you've never had a night of uninterrupted, restful sleep, you may not even know that you're missing it.

LISTEN TO THE BEAT OF YOUR CIRCADIAN RHYTHMS

We live in accordance with our circadian rhythms, the physical, mental, and behavioral changes that follow a 24-hour cycle. These natural processes, which affect most living things (including plants), respond primarily to light and dark. According to our natural body clock, we should be spending about a third of our time sleeping—that's about seven to nine hours out of every 24. Only one out of three Americans is getting enough sleep today.

THE LINK BETWEEN SLEEPING AND EATING

There is mounting evidence linking lack of sleep with obesity. At least one reason for this is that lack of sleep affects the production of the hormones that control hunger and satiety.

Ghrelin stimulates appetite, and people who are sleep-deprived have been shown to have higher levels of ghrelin than those who get seven to nine hours of sleep.

Leptin is the hormone that helps to regulate energy balance by inhibiting hunger, which, in turn, diminishes fat storage.

The problem is that when your sleep is out of whack, so are those hormones. Sleep deprivation increases ghrelin levels while also reducing leptin levels in the blood, signaling to your brain that your energy supply is limited so that the brain, in turn, tells your gastrointestinal tract that you are hungry!

That's bad enough, but since you're sleep-deprived, your energy level really is low (but not because you need to eat). Therefore, you crave foods that are going to raise your blood sugar levels—just as you do when you hit the office candy machine at three o'clock in the afternoon when you need a pick-me-up. So you go for the sugary carbs, which are exactly what you don't need when what you do need is to sleep.

WHAT'S GOOD FOR YOUR BODY IS GOOD FOR YOUR MOUTH

According to the National Heart, Lung, and Blood Institute, it is a common myth "that people can learn to get by on little sleep with no negative effects. However, research shows that getting enough quality sleep at the right times is vital for mental health, physical health, quality of life, and safety." Lack of sleep is linked to heart disease, kidney disease, high blood pressure, diabetes, stroke, obesity, and depression, not to mention an increased chance of injury, falls, and broken bones.

And your oral health is equally dependent on sleep, because your mouth's self-cleaning system, including your saliva, has evolved to work in accordance with your circadian rhythms.

Staying up late often means eating and drinking late as well. That's fine and fun once in a while, but we need to give our oral cleaning system time to do its job by giving ourselves enough sleep. Think of it like rebooting your computer. Shutting down and restarting the operating system solves many problems such as slow processing or freezing.

> *In fact, sometimes physical symptoms of poor sleep show up first in your mouth.*

According to the American Academy of Medical Orthodontics, a number of studies have shown that the risk of developing gum disease and inflammation is higher among people who are sleep-deprived.

Poor sleep and stress often go hand in hand, and the symptoms often overlap. When you're stressed or sleep-deprived (or both), you may be clenching and/or grinding your teeth, sleeping with your mouth open, and experiencing dry mouth. In addition to exacerbating dry mouth, sleeping with your mouth open can disturb the balance of oral bacteria, which in turn can also disrupt your oral microbiome and put you at higher risk for inflammation.

Pain and clicking can come from your temporomandibular joint (TMJ), which helps you move your jaw when you're speaking and chewing. TMJ disorder comes from clenching your jaw and/or grinding your teeth—also signs of stress—and straining the muscles around your face. Grinding also wears away your enamel and can cause jaw problems and/or headaches.

Finally, it's important to keep your tongue lightly resting against your upper palate. We'll be talking more about this in the next chapter, but poor tongue posture can lead to a variety of problems including a stiff neck and uneven teeth.

SIGNS OF POOR SLEEP

THE TROUBLE WITH SNORING

You snore when and if air cannot flow freely through your airway as you breathe in and out during sleep. You might then wake up gasping for air, which obviously interrupts your sleep and can cause your body to go into "fight or flight" mode (because it senses that you are in danger), which has been associated with high blood pressure and other stress-related problems.

In addition, while all snoring is related to breathing problems, it can be a sign that you are suffering from obstructive sleep apnea (OSA), a condition that causes your breathing to stop and start while you are sleeping because your upper airway relaxes and collapses, which can actually be life-threatening. When you have sleep apnea, you snore because your brain senses that you're not getting enough oxygen, and briefly rouses you from sleep so that you can reopen your airway. You may not even realize that you've been woken, but there are symptoms you can look for if you suspect you have a problem.

OSA used to be thought of as a male ailment, but it is increasingly recognized as a female disease as well. Surprisingly, studies have revealed significant gender disparities in symptoms, diagnosis, repercussions, and treatment. Women have less severe OSA, a lower apnea-hypopnea score, and shorter apneas and hypopneas,*

---

* **Apnea:** An apnea is a complete cessation of airflow for at least 10 seconds.
Hypopnea: A hypopnea is a partial reduction in airflow for at least 10 seconds, accompanied by a decrease in oxygen saturation or an arousal from sleep.

to name a few. They also have lower rates of prevalence and fewer correct diagnoses. According to the studies, hormones play a role in some gender-related variances, with the prevalence decreasing with age. It has also been observed that, despite the lower prevalence and severity of OSA in women, the consequences are comparable or worse for the same severity.

TYPICAL SYMPTOMS FROM SLEEP APNEA:

- Loud snoring
- Gasping for air during sleep
- Grinding your teeth
- Awakening with dry mouth
- Morning headaches
- Insomnia
- Excessive sleepiness during the day
- Difficulty focusing or paying attention
- Irritability
- Chronic stress
- Mouth breathing

SYMPTOMS FROM A SLEEP STUDY WITH ALL FEMALE SUBJECTS:

- Loud snoring
- Episodes in which you stop breathing during sleep—which would be reported by another person
- Gasping for air during sleep
- Awakening with a dry mouth
- Morning headache
- Difficulty staying asleep, known as insomnia
- Excessive daytime sleepiness, known as hypersomnia

If you've noticed any of these symptoms, or if your partner tells you that you stopped breathing while you were asleep, you should consult a healthcare professional to determine if it is really sleep apnea and, if so, to discuss your treatment options.

TREATING OBSTRUCTIVE SLEEP APNEA

Dr. Maria Sokolina, a Diplomate of the American Board of Dental Sleep Medicine, has shared her broad knowledge of some of the treatments and management options for sleep apnea, which range from simple lifestyle changes to actual plastic surgery. It would be up to you and your doctor to determine which, if any, of these would be either appropriate or necessary for you.

THE CPAP MACHINE is probably the most common form of management. It requires you to wear a mask and delivers pressurized air that prevents your airway from collapsing.

THE INSPIRE IMPLANT involves the implantation of a small device that is activated by remote control when you go to bed, to keep your airway open while you sleep.

AN ORAL APPLIANCE is removable, and fits over your upper and lower teeth when you sleep to move your lower jaw forward, preventing your tongue from obstructing your airway, and toning the muscles of your soft palate.

SURGICAL OPTIONS INCLUDE:

- Orthodontic surgery to move both your upper and lower jaw to open your airway.
- Inserting a mini appliance to expand your palate.
- Plastic surgery to correct a blockage in the area behind the soft palate.
- Surgery to reduce the small bony structures inside your nose (called turbinates) to correct a deviated septum, and/or endoscopic surgery for sinus inflammation.

Additional adjunct therapies could include:

- Physical therapy for the tongue, lips, and soft palate to encourage nose (as opposed to mouth) breathing.
- eXiteOSA daytime therapy to strengthen weak tongue muscles.
- A Bongo Rx machine for people with mild to moderate sleep apnea who naturally breathe through their nose.
- Nasal irrigation and/or dilation to expand the airway.
- Mouth taping to promote nose breathing (see below).
- Lifestyle changes, including weight loss and decreased alcohol consumption.

THE NIGHTLY GRIND

You may not even realize that you're grinding your teeth, especially if you do it while you're sleeping. Many people don't know it until their dentist sees signs of worn enamel. It's generally just written off as a sign of stress, but 33 to 54 percent of people with sleep apnea also grind their teeth, suggesting that there may be an association between the two conditions. While it isn't clear how the two are related, one theory is that the grinding may be a way to wake yourself up when you stop breathing. It is also common among people with GERD (gastrointestinal reflux disease) and has been associated with certain medications, including amphetamines, antipsychotics, and antidepressants, as well as with cocaine and ecstasy.

If you do notice wear in your own mouth, if you have receding gums that could be exacerbated by grinding, or if you wake up with headaches in the morning, you should talk to your dentist about the possibility that you are a night-grinder and what you can do about it. This could also mean that you have sleep apnea without being aware of it.

Tip: If you determine that you are grinding your teeth, ask your dentist whether you are a candidate for a night guard to wear when sleeping.

TRY TAPING YOUR MOUTH

I know this may sound radical if not actually punitive, but I really urge you to try it. I've been doing it for a few years now. Sleep experts do not all agree on the benefits of mouth-taping, but I have found it extremely helpful. The taping of your lips is to practice keeping the mouth closed in a relaxed way while sleeping.

Place the mouth tape over your mouth for about 10 minutes, and then work up to 20–30 minutes or so over the next couple of days. When you feel your body is used to breathing through the nose, use the mouth tape for the night.

Here are a couple examples of benefits for your health when you breathe through your nose:

- Improves the quality of your sleep because breathing through your nose puts you into a state of rest and digest rather than fight or flight.
- Helps to prevent sleep apnea.
- Improves oral health because it is keeping the mouth moist while you are sleeping.
- Helps to stabilize the pH balance of the oral microbiome.

Since I've been doing it, I've come to appreciate how much nose breathing contributes to my general well-being. When I first heard about it, I tried taping my mouth for a while before I went to sleep, and as I got used to it, I started keeping the tape on all night. At the same time, after becoming familiar with Anders Olsson's *Conscious Breathing*, I made it a point to become aware of my breathing habits and discovered how I could take control of my breathing to control my stress. In the next chapter you can read more about breathing.

> Research has shown that you can't actually "catch up" on lost sleep. According to Dr. Yelena Tumashova, a sleep medicine specialist at Advocate Lutheran General Hospital in Park Ridge, Illinois, "Changing your sleep habits on the weekends can actually be detrimental for your health as you are changing your sleep architecture and circadian rhythms..."

ARE YOU READY TO MAKE NEW HABITS?

If you're ready to make some new habits that will improve your oral and overall health by improving your sleep, here are a few suggestions to get you started.

BEFORE GOING TO BED HABITS:

- Finish your last meal at least two hours—and preferably three—before you go to bed, because your mouth needs that time to clean itself and also because eating is likely to boost your energy, which is not what you need to do just before bedtime.
- Start preparing for bed by turning off the bright lights in your bedroom.
- Don't drink coffee close to bedtime if you know it's going to keep you from sleeping.

- If you take medications or supplements, consider whether taking them a bit earlier—or, if possible, in the morning rather than the evening—would prevent them from interfering with your sleep.

BEDROOM HABITS:

- Keep your bedroom as cool as is comfortable for you.
- Make sure to keep your bedroom a special place, mainly for sleeping if possible.
- Make it as dark as you can (especially during the summer, when it's lighter for longer).
- Declutter your bedroom.

GOING TO BED HABITS:

- Go to bed and get up at the same time every day of the week, including weekends. Set an alarm if you need to, but don't just roll over and go back to sleep!
- Don't let your to-do list get in the way of your sleep. Keep a pad and pencil by your bed to write down ideas that pop randomly into your head when you ought to be sleeping.
- Keep a simple sleep journal. Each morning, write down the number of hours you slept, how easy or difficult it was to fall asleep, and how rested you felt upon waking. This would be a great way to learn more about yourself as well as providing information to share with a healthcare professional.
- Practice nose breathing by mouth-taping at night.
  - Find a tape that works for you.
  - Start small with a lighter, smaller piece of tape.

SUMMARY OF CHAPTER 5

1   Sleep and oral health are interconnected. The way we sleep affects our breath, oral microbiome, and the skin on our face.

2   Poor sleep can lead to gum disease, inflammation, dry mouth, teeth grinding, and jaw problems.

3   Snoring can be a sign of interrupted sleep and breathing problems. It can also indicate a more severe condition called obstructive sleep apnea or OSA, where breathing repeatedly stops and starts during sleep. Symptoms of OSA include loud snoring, gasping for air, morning headaches, and excessive daytime sleepiness.

4   Maintain a consistent sleep schedule, and avoid stimulating activities, bright lights, and heavy meals before bed. Practice nose breathing, create a sleep-friendly environment, and avoid caffeine, alcohol, and medications close to bedtime. Keep a sleep journal and consult a healthcare professional for any sleep-related issues.

SLEEP: HABITS WORKSHEET

CONNECT

Write down your top 3 aspirations for your life

Example: I want to improve my overall health

_____

_____

_____

_____

_____

CURATE

What habits do you want to practice? List a few habits that you would consider trying as a way to reach your aspirations. Remember to identify habits that are small, doable, and practical (realistic). Also favor habits that can be integrated into your existing daily routines.

Examples: More consistent sleeping, 7–8 hours per night. Go to bed at the same time each night.

_____

_____

_____

_____

_____

_____

CREATE

Now, when you are set on what new habits you want to commit to, consider the context of your life and make sure you remove all reasons to say no and make it as easy as you can to say yes!

Example: I commit to practicing nose breathing by using mouth tape every night.

What? _____

_____

When? _____

How? _____

_____

I commit to: _____

_____

_____

_____

_____

_____

_____

CELEBRATE

Be your own cheerleader! Every day you practice the habit, you will celebrate with a pat on the shoulder and say "Well done!"

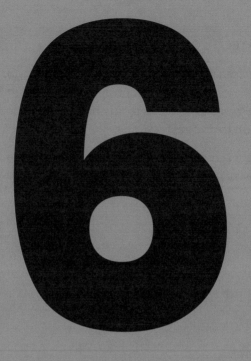

CHAPTER

6

HOW TO
BREATHE EASY

BREATHE

[*andas*]

I know, I know—breathing is automatic. It's not something you think about, except when you're "out of breath," for whatever reason. But just because it's automatic doesn't mean it's out of your control. Nor does it mean that you're breathing as well as you might be. And your mouth can let you know when you need to change the way you breathe.

Many years ago, when I was a professional golfer and under pressure in competitions, I would step up to hit a ball with my heart pounding in my chest. Focusing on my breathing would help me slow down and do what I had trained for. But even then, I didn't really consider how my breathing was affecting my ability to function at peak performance.

It wasn't until I was given the book *Breath* by science journalist James Nestor that I truly came to understand how much the way we breathe has to do with our overall health. As Nestor said, and I now appreciate, "No matter what we eat, how much we exercise, how resilient our genes are, how skinny or young or wise we are—none of it will matter unless we're breathing correctly." Coming to that understanding has been life-changing for me.

We spend a lot of time and money on supplements, gym memberships, and fancy diets, but the best thing we can do for our health and happiness is to pay more attention to how we breathe—and it doesn't cost a cent!

HOW DO YOU BREATHE?

Answering that question probably isn't as easy as you would have thought because most of us breathe without really thinking about it. According to the Canadian Lung Association, we breathe in and out approximately 25,000 times a day, so if we had to think about it, we wouldn't have much time left to think about anything else! But I do want you to think about it for the next couple of minutes. Indulge me!

Take a few breaths and notice what happens. Do your shoulders move up? Does your belly expand? When you breathe out are you blowing all the air out of your lungs or is some of it still left? Make a note of what you've observed and then return to your normal way of breathing. Is your mouth open? Is your belly rising and falling? Is your tongue relaxed? Make a note of these observations and read on to find out what it all means.

> **66**
>
> When we breathe right, we can control our bodies in ways that we never thought possible.
>
> **—James Nestor**
>
> **99**

In his book *Breath: The New Science of a Lost Art*, James Nestor discusses the connection between breathing and jaw development and beyond. He writes about a personal experiment he did with Anders Olsson at a lab at Stanford, where during the experiment they alternated between breathing exclusively through their noses and exclusively through their mouths. The purpose of this experiment was to understand the potential physiological and health effects of nasal breathing versus mouth breathing.

Nestor also explores the impact of modern lifestyle factors, such as processed diets and changes in oral posture, on the proper growth and development of the jaws.

The author has done a great job, to my mind, with his research, and writes in a highly flowing style. I couldn't stop reading it.

ARE YOU A MOUTH-BREATHER?

In the previous chapter we talked about snoring, teeth grinding, and other signs of sleep disruption, all of which are caused by, amongst other things, breathing through your mouth. Studies have also shown that mouth breathing can either lead to or worsen sleep apnea by increasing airway collapse or nasal congestion.

But, again, breathing is a full-time job, and mouth breathing can lead to a number of problems that are not specifically related to sleep. These include:

• Headaches
• Sore throat and cold symptoms
• Inflamed gums
• Bad breath
• Increased risk of cavities
• Asthma
• Digestive disturbances, including gas, upset stomach, and acid reflux

When you breathe through your mouth, your mouth dries out, meaning that you have less saliva available for cleaning. And, to make matters worse, you are bypassing the process by which the tiny hairs in your nose, called cilia, filter out allergens, dust particles, viruses, and bacteria, and prevent them from entering your body.

> ❝
>
> ## When I learned how to breathe, I learned how to live.
>
> **—Anders Olsson, founder of Conscious Breathing**
>
> ❞

THE NOSE KNOWS

While mouth breathing can create all kinds of health problems, breathing through your nose does just the opposite. The benefits are manifold:

- As mentioned above, the hairs in your nose filter out dust, allergens, and pollen and prevent them from entering your lungs.

- Nose breathing warms and moisturizes the air you take in, bringing it to body temperature and making it easier for your lungs to use.

- Breathing through your nose stimulates your parasympathetic nervous system to put you into a calming state of rest and digest.

- When you breathe through your nose (but not your mouth), your sinuses produce nitric oxide, a vasodilator, which opens up the blood vessels. This, in turn, improves oxygen circulation in the body.

So, once again, what's good for your mouth is good for your body.

EXPLORING NITRIC OXIDE AND ITS HEALTH BENEFITS THROUGH NOSE BREATHING

I've been hooked on nose breathing as part of my everyday (and nightly) well-being. I've been taping my mouth while I sleep to encourage breathing through my nose exclusively, and I truly feel better every morning waking up since I started doing this.

There is one benefit to nose breathing that I did not know about until recently. When you breathe in and out through your nose, you produce and inhale nitric oxide. NO is produced inside our sinuses and travels through our sinuses' airways all the way to our lungs.

I first heard about NO when I listened to Mark Hyman's interview with Dr. Louis Ignarro on his podcast, *Food Farmacy*. In 1998 Dr. Ignarro was awarded the Nobel Prize in Medicine and Physiology, jointly with Robert F. Furchgott and Ferrid Murad, for their work on the role of nitric oxide as a signaling molecule in the cardiovascular system. That's how innovative NO research has been! So much of what we know about its practical application has only been discovered in the last few decades.

A very basic explanation of NO

NO goes to the lungs; it relaxes the bronchi,* so they widen. It also works as a vasodilator, which means that it relaxes the inner muscles of your blood vessels, causing the vessels to widen. What happens then is that it increases blood flow and lowers blood pressure.

This lowering of blood pressure is linked to several health benefits, such as lower stress, better sleep regulation, reduced anxiety and greater relaxation. It's also linked to a longer lifespan and better immune function. The brain has ten times more nitric oxide than any other part of the body. Are you sold yet?

One of the things that makes NO so special is that it's a gas that acts as a neurotransmitter, sending signals between nerve cells in the body. Doing this has a big impact on our cardiovascular and circulatory systems.

Nitric oxide is formed in our bodies either naturally or as a result of eating foods high in nitrate, L-arginine, and L-citrulline.

When nitrate intake is from food, nitrate is converted to nitrite (NO_2)—primarily in the back of the tongue—which is then transformed to nitric oxide (NO) in the upper gastrointestinal system.

I hope you're sitting there thinking: So, how do I make sure I'm producing more NO?

Well, there's **exercise**:
- People with more sedentary lifestyles (sorry to say!) have been shown to have lower NO levels, while people who do more

---

* **Bronchi** (singular: bronchus) are the major air passages in the respiratory system that carry air from the trachea (windpipe) into the lungs.

physical activity—even just walking—are shown to produce more NO.

And there's **food**:
- Food sources include leafy greens and beets! Time for some borscht!

THE SKY TECHNIQUE

SKY stands for Sudarshan Kriya Yoga, and the SKY technique is a form of meditation that increases nitric oxide production. Try it for yourself. Sit comfortably in a quiet place and breathe through your nose for a count of four. Then hold your breath for a count of four, and slowly release it to a count of eight.

Repeat this simple exercise and see how much better you feel. You have just boosted your nitric oxide levels.

BELLY BREATHING FOR BETTER HEALTH

Belly breathing is simply a less fancy way of saying that you should be breathing into your diaphragm. Your diaphragm is a muscle at the base of your lungs. When you breath in, it contracts, making more room in your chest cavity for your lungs to expand, and when you exhale, it relaxes, moves upward in your chest cavity, and forces the air out of your lungs. That kind of breathing activates your parasympathetic nervous system, which can help to lower your heart rate and reduce your blood pressure.

TO PRACTICE BELLY BREATHING:

- Sit in a chair with your knees bent and your shoulders, head, and neck relaxed.

- Place one hand on your upper chest and the other just below your rib cage.

- Breathe in slowly through your nose so that your stomach pushes against your hand. Keep the hand on your chest as still as possible.

- Tighten your stomach muscles so that your stomach moves back in while you exhale through pursed lips, again keeping your upper chest as still as possible.

The more you practice this exercise, the easier and more automatic belly breathing will become. The stresses of modern life keep too many of us in a stressed-out state of "fight or flight" too often and for too long. The more we can relax, lower our heart rate, and reduce our blood pressure, the better off we'll be.

WHERE DO YOU KEEP YOUR TONGUE?

Yes, I know, you keep it in your mouth, but *where* in your mouth is the question.

Ideally, when you are relaxed, your tongue should press lightly against the roof of your mouth just behind your front teeth. Your mouth should be closed and your teeth slightly parted.

Your tongue is a strong muscle whose posture can impact other parts of your body, including not only your mouth but your eyes, nose, head, neck, and shoulders. It can contribute to sleep apnea, vision problems, bad posture, and, of course, tooth damage.

If you rest your tongue on the bottom of your mouth or up against your teeth, it is in the wrong position. Resting your tongue on the bottom of your mouth can cause neck and jaw pain, and putting pressure on your teeth can cause them to shift over time, causing teeth grinding, as well as increasing decay.

TRY THIS TONGUE POSTURE EXERCISE

1 Place the tip of your tongue against the roof of your mouth behind your front teeth.

___

2 Use suction to pull all of your tongue flat against the roof of your mouth. (This may be difficult at first. Keep at it.)

___

3 Close your mouth.

___

4 Hold your tongue in that position, breathing as normally as possible.

To challenge yourself even more, open your mouth and see how much and for how long you can hold your tongue in place.

Do this as often as you can for as long as you can. Your tongue is a muscle and needs to be strengthened through training, just like any other muscle.

The following suggestions for better breathing are inspired by Anders Olsson, author of *Conscious Breathing: Discover the Power of Your Breath*.

Olsson argues that we can use our breathing to improve our ability to manage our thoughts and emotions. As with any other strategy, you need knowledge, the right tools, and intentionality to make it happen. However, since we always breathe, you can practice these seven advised breathing techniques whenever you like. After your first deep, slow, through-the-nose, rhythmic small and calm breath, you will most likely feel different.

1 NOSE
In the airways leading to the lungs, the air is warmed, moisturized, and purified. You should focus on inhaling and exhaling through your nose if possible.

2 DIAPHRAGM
Our breathing should reach into the lower part of our lungs, using the diaphragm. Did you know that the diaphragm and the heart are the only muscles in your body that never rest?

3 SLOW
Healthy breathing should occur at a rate of no more than six to twelve breaths per minute. What rate are you breathing at?

4 SMALL BREATHS
Many of us have a tendency to take big, fast breaths. When you breathe, you inhale oxygen and exhale carbon dioxide. Excessive breathing may lead to low levels of carbon dioxide in your blood, which can cause dizziness and many of the other symptoms that you can feel when you hyperventilate.

5 POSTURE
Your posture affects your breathing. Put a hand on your chest and one on your stomach and take a small breath. Notice where the

air goes. Now, do the same in an intentionally erect position and notice if there is any difference in how deep the breath is.

6 RHYTHMIC
Check in on your breathing throughout the day. Are you holding your breath while working on the computer?

7 QUIETLY
When we sniff, snore, sigh, or clear our throats, we breathe. These breaths are very ineffective, which creates unnecessary stress on our bodies.

ARE YOU READY TO MAKE NEW HABITS?

BREATHING HABITS
- Go over the seven suggestions for better breathing and see what you might want to focus on to improve your breathing and well-being.

BREATHING EXERCISES
- To practice belly breathing, see page 122.

BOOST YOUR NO
- Use the SKY technique.
- Start a new habit to include more NO-boosting vegetables.

TONGUE PRACTICE
- Try the tongue positioning exercise described above.
- Consciously check out the position of your tongue throughout the day.

SUMMARY OF CHAPTER 6

1   Breathing through your nose has numerous benefits, such as filtering dust, allergens, and pollen, moisturizing and warming the air, stimulating nitric oxide production that has positive effects on your arteries, and more.

2   Practice diaphragmatic breathing, i.e. slow and low (down in your belly) breaths. This activates the parasympathetic nervous system, helping to lower the heart rate and blood pressure within a couple of breaths.

3   Maintain proper tongue positioning. Your tongue should be resting lightly against the roof of your mouth, behind the front teeth (not pushing on the teeth). This helps you maintain a wide palate and breathe better.

BREATHE: HABITS WORKSHEET

CONNECT

Write down your top 3 aspirations for your life

Example: I want to improve my overall health

_____

_____

_____

_____

_____

CURATE

What habits do you want to practice? List a few habits that you would consider trying as a way to reach your aspirations. Remember to identify habits that are small, doable, and practical (realistic). Also favor habits that can be integrated into your existing daily routines.

Examples: Practice nose breathing. Morning meditation routine with focus on my breathing.

_____

_____

_____

_____

_____

_____

CREATE

Now, when you are set on which or what new habits you want to commit to, consider the context of your life and make sure you remove all reasons to say no and make it as easy as you can to say yes!

Example: I commit to practicing nose breathing by using mouth tape every night.

What? _____

_____

When? _____

How? _____

_____

I commit to: _____

_____

_____

_____

_____

_____

_____

CELEBRATE

Be your own cheerleader! Every day you practice the habit, you will celebrate with a pat on the shoulder and say "Well done!"

CHAPTER 7

MOVE YOUR BODY, MOVE YOUR MIND

MOVE

[*rörelse*]

n addition to optimizing your way of eating, sleeping, and breathing, your oral and overall health depend on *moving*. Please note that I have intentionally *not* used the term "exercise," which for many people not only has a negative connotation but also refers to something that requires a degree of physical or athletic ability.

What I'm talking about is something different. No matter our level of physical ability, we can all find ways to move our bodies and live a more active lifestyle.

Mike Young, a performance and fitness coach who holds a Ph.D. in kinesiology, compares an active lifestyle to a form of over-the-counter medicine that has no side effects and requires no prescription. In a TEDx talk he gave in 2021, he indicated that an active lifestyle was proven to treat many common diseases ranging from Alzheimer's to type 2 diabetes, as well as anxiety and stress.

But, as with most things in life, it's not just the physical aspect of movement that's important. I'd also like to invite you to move your *mind*—to keep it open to new ideas and to incorporate mindfulness and stress relief into your daily habits.

You might believe that moving your mind and your body are two separate aspects of your existence. I would rather argue that they are intertwined. I suggest that we think better when we move, and our desire to move our bodies starts in our minds. At the same time, the arguments we make up for not moving our bodies start in our minds as well.

It is a well-known fact that people are more likely to act themselves into new ways of thinking rather than think themselves into new ways of acting.

I would argue that if you get up and move, it will also help shape how you think about things. When I have a problem, I find that getting my body moving and "walking it off" really helps.

At this point, there is basically no argument about the fact that chronic stress can have a serious negative effect on your physical health. According to the American Psychological Association, "Stress involves changes affecting nearly every system of the body, influencing how people feel and behave." They also say that, "By causing mind-body changes, stress contributes directly to psychological and physiological disorders and diseases and affects mental and physical health, reducing quality of life."

Conversely, any activity that helps you to destress or unwind will have a positive impact on your overall health, and, thereby, on your oral health as well. We all need to move our bodies *and* our minds every day. And we have far more opportunities than we think to do that, even when we believe we don't have the time. While writing this book, for example, I took a lot of walks to help me develop my thoughts, open my mind, and tap into my creativity.

> What is good exercise? The kind that gets done!

REASONS TO KEEP MOVING

One of the most essential things you can do for your health is engage in regular physical activity and move your body.

I know you might not be as likely to get up and move as I am. However, it is my firm belief that you don't need to start training to become an athlete; just start moving in your everyday life. Find what works for you, and make sure it's something that gives you pleasure and a reason to spend time with friends, colleagues, and family. Why not try something new, or revisit an activity you used to like doing when you were younger?

Maybe you will be inspired when you hear that physical activity may enhance your mental health, help you control your weight, lower your risk of disease, strengthen your bones and muscles, and increase your ability to complete everyday tasks.

And this goes for any age group!

> **People who are regularly active have a stronger sense of purpose, and they experience more gratitude, love, and hope. They feel more connected to their communities, and are less likely to suffer from loneliness or become depressed.**
>
> —Kelly McGonigal, *The Joy of Movement*

If you need even more reasons to start moving, here are some for you:

MOVEMENT HAS A POSITIVE EFFECT ON YOUR DIGESTION

Movement can have a positive impact on the body by increasing endorphins, lowering stress, improving blood flow, and accelerating metabolism. On the other hand, a lack of physical activity might be detrimental to your digestive system. Most forms of movement, including yoga and cardio activities, can help with digestion.

PHYSICAL ACTIVITY INCREASES YOUR ENERGY LEVEL

It is widely accepted that regular physical activity can improve your muscle strength and boost your endurance. Exercise delivers oxygen and nutrients to your tissues and helps your cardiovascular system work more efficiently. And when your heart and lung health improve, you have more energy to tackle daily chores.

MOVEMENT INCREASES BRAIN POWER

Swedish physician and psychiatrist Anders Hansen is well known for his work in the fields of fitness and mental health. Hansen discusses the effects of physical movement on cognitive capacities and mental health in his book *The Real Happy Pill: Power Up Your Brain by Moving Your Body.*

Regular physical activity, according to Hansen, has a dramatic effect on the brain. He claims that exercise causes the brain to produce more chemicals such as endorphins and serotonin which promote better mood, reduce anxiety, and improve cognitive performance. Personally, I find that when I feel unmotivated, getting up and moving around can quickly get me back on track.

MOVING IMPROVES SLEEPING

Although those who have a hard time sleeping might want to avoid intense activity right before bedtime, Charlene Gamaldo, MD, medical director of the Johns Hopkins Center for Sleep at

Howard County Medical Center, says that, based on available studies, "We have solid evidence that exercise does, in fact, help you fall asleep more quickly and improves sleep quality." There's still some debate as to what time of day you should exercise. I encourage people to listen to their bodies to see how well they sleep in response to when they work out.

MOVING IMPROVES YOUR MOOD

Maybe you feel the same happiness I do when you are dancing. That is an example of how we can improve our mood by moving. You've probably heard of a "runner's high," even if you haven't experienced it yourself. That's because movement increases the release of "happy hormones" (serotonin, dopamine, endorphins, and oxytocin) in your body.

THE LINK BETWEEN ORAL HEALTH AND PHYSICAL ACTIVITY

As I keep saying, what's good for your body is good for your mouth, and research has shown that people who are more active are also more likely to have better oral health than those who are sedentary.

A LOWER RISK OF GUM DISEASE

Exercise is considered to produce anti-inflammatory effects that are beneficial to the body. This, in turn, can help lessen the severity of certain chronic illnesses, which can ultimately have a favorable influence on general and oral health.

Of course, exercise alone isn't enough to guarantee good oral health. A study published in the *British Dental Journal* found that almost half of elite endurance athletes suffered from untreated tooth decay and showed signs of gum disease. Clearly this wasn't

> # DID YOU KNOW?
>
> Moderate movement has been shown to increase production of your saliva proteins and, therefore, provide more protection against inflammation and gum disease. According to a study published in the March 21, 2019 issue of *Frontiers in Physiology*, "Physical activity was associated as a potential tool for a reduction of periodontal disease prevalence."

due to a lack of movement! The reason, the study concluded, was because "they often refuel with high-acid drinks, gels and energy bars—all of which can weaken tooth enamel and damage teeth due to high sugar content and acidity." So, it's best to avoid sugar and rehydrate with plain water as necessary.

A POSITIVE EFFECT ON THE ORAL MICROBIOME

"Exercise promotes a healthy and diverse oral microbiome," according to a recent research review that includes the following key findings:

- Moderate (*lagom*) regular exercise increases salivary production in older people.
- Moderate exercise can reduce the risk of infections by increasing the levels of salivary cystines, which play an essential role in tooth remineralization and protection.

While the benefits of exercise for gut bacteria and overall health are already well established, new research shows that exercise-induced physical stress also promotes a healthy and more diverse oral microbiome.

That said, the opposite could be said about the effects of mental stress (or distress). Stress reduces saliva flow and increases the acidity in your mouth, which can lead to a higher risk of cavities and inflammation. That a side-effect of physical exercise is stress reduction means that it is also valuable for your oral health.

EVERYTHING WORKS BOTH WAYS

If physical activity promotes oral and overall health, it's also true, of course, that problems such as inflammation or pain in your mouth, your body, or both can easily prevent you from achieving peak performance in athletics, or any kind of activity that requires movement, strength, and coordination.

TIPS FOR CREATIVE WALKING

When I read that Steve Jobs believed that his most creative ideas occurred while he was walking and that he often met with staff while walking around, I was inspired to incorporate walking into my own writing process and to ask other people to join me.

Be aware: If you want to have a productive "walking meeting," make sure the other person is both willing and able to join you. Move at a pace that allows you both to remain cool, calm, and creative. Remember, this is a meeting, not a marathon.

Once your eyes are open to new possibilities, you'll begin to see them everywhere. That is as true for opportunities to increase physical activity as it is for virtually every other aspect of your life.

Moving can mean many different things to many people: tending the garden, walking the dog, going for a jog, running up and down the stairs, running after the kids or grandkids, walking to the bus stop. Keep your mind open to what is possible! Just thinking about how to start something new is, in itself, a way of moving your mind instead of your feet. We all need to find time for both.

LOCATION, LOCATION, LOCATION!

Many studies have shown that contact with nature promotes human health. Being out in nature has been found to be relaxing, which decreases stress and protects against inflammation, which is beneficial to your overall and oral health. Therefore, if you spend time moving outdoors, you may be doing yourself an even bigger favor than if you spent that same time exercising in a gym.

TAKE TIME TO RECHARGE

The Sanford Health Initiative defines the term "recharge" as "sleeping or relaxing to restore energy." To recharge, you can try the following activities besides sleeping:

• Practicing a low-intensity exercise like yoga
• Journaling
• Reading
• Meditation/breathing
• Putting together a puzzle

As a competitive golfer, I always loved the focus involved in the repetitive movement of hitting balls at the driving range. For me, it is still extremely meditative and stress-relieving. I urge you to find your own favorite way to achieve the stress-relief we all need from time to time.

The very act of repetition allows you to be mindful and thoughtful, and can be an incredibly powerful way to boost your mental and overall health. It could be something creative, like drawing, painting, or reading. Maybe for you it's gardening, knitting, or cooking. Just keep your eyes open for opportunities to focus and find mental stillness.

MEDITATION

Way back when, in the early 1990s, I was fortunate enough to be exposed to meditation when my husband and I went to meditation training at the Brahma Kumaris center in Stockholm, Sweden. Since then, I've used meditation to recharge and reset when I feel the need. And I do feel the need a lot!

Instead of me telling you what meditation is or can be, I'm quoting Brahma Kumaris in this beautiful statement: "Meditation is the journey inwards, a journey of self-discovery or, in fact, re-discovery. Meditation is time taken for quiet reflection and silence, away from the hustle and bustle of daily living. Taking time out enables us to come back to a centered place of being."

The practice of meditation is diverse and very personal. It can be tailored to the individual's preferences and needs. It is an exploration of the mind and inner experience. Finding your unique way of meditating is part of the journey, as I see it. There are plenty of meditation techniques, styles, and "gurus" out there to choose from.

I hope that starting with the following basic general steps can be an inspiration for you to try something new, or a revisit for those who have meditated before. These steps provide a framework to initiate your journey, but remember that they are not set in stone.

Meditation is a personal and continuously evolving practice.

1 SETTLING THE MIND
Here you are creating a calm and focused state. I suggest that you start with sitting in a comfortable chair or on the floor on a pillow, whatever works for you. Now it's time to focus on your breathing in and out of the nose. This will calm you down after just a few breaths.

2 CULTIVATING AWARENESS
Here is where you practice observing your thoughts, sensations, and emotions without judgment or attachment. Let your thoughts come and go, passing through.

3 SUSTAINING THE PRACTICE
Start small (really small, like a minute or two) and build as you go. Cultivate awareness and gently let your thoughts pass by. They will probably keep coming, so focus on letting them go instead of trying not to have any thoughts at all.

HYDRATING

Proper hydration is a popular topic these days, particularly in conjunction with physical activity, and there is some disagreement about whether sports drinks are more beneficial than water when exercising. I believe—and studies have shown—that unless you're engaging in prolonged, intense exercise, basically on a professional level, it's better to stick with water than it is to consume sugary sports drinks.

Studies have shown that energy drinks can cause damage to the teeth. In fact, constant drinking of any kind when you are exercising can impact your saliva and, therefore, the bacteria in your mouth, which, in turn, can increase your risk of developing cavities and gum disease.

ARE YOU READY TO MAKE NEW HABITS?

There's a right way and a wrong way to do just about everything, and not all behaviors associated with exercise or movement are healthy for you.

AFTER-DINNER WALK

I challenge you to incorporate a walk after dinner as much as the weather permits, to give you time to end the day on a "high note," work through "stuff" from the past day, and also give your digestion a boost.

SMALL MEALS (AKA SNACKS)

Just because you've been moving more than usual doesn't mean you have permission to snack. Make sure you eat a healthy, health-promoting meal that will sustain you until it's time for your next meal.

BREATHING

Mouth breathing during exercise can dry out your mouth, which will then affect your oral bacteria and potentially lead to cavities and gum disease. Consciously breathing in and out through your nose when you are pushing yourself while exercising can help you get through it, because your breathing slows down.

STAYING SAFE

If you're engaging in an activity that could cause injury, wear the proper protective gear, such as mouth guard, helmet, or even shin guards.

RECHARGING

Find ways to relax and regain your strength. Incorporate breathing exercises or meditation into your daily routine as much as you can fit it in. You can always start very small with only a couple of minutes of meditation, for example (see page 140).

HYDRATING

Choose wisely what you drink when you are exercising. Water might be the best choice, rather than sugary sports drinks.

SUMMARY OF CHAPTER 7

1   Stress reduces saliva flow and increases the acidity in your mouth, which can lead to a higher risk of cavities and inflammation.

2   Exercise promotes a healthy and diverse oral microbiome.

3   Moderate movement has been shown to increase the production of salivary proteins and, therefore, provide more protection against inflammation and gum disease.

4   Moving can mean many different activities, such as tending the garden, walking the dog, going for a jog, running up and down the stairs, running after kids, or walking to the bus stop. Just thinking about how to start something new is a way to move your mind instead of your feet.

5   Open your eyes to new possibilities and look for opportunities to increase physical activity.

MOVE: HABITS WORKSHEET

CONNECT

Write down your top 3 aspirations for your life

Example: I want to improve my overall health

_____

_____

_____

_____

CURATE

What habits do you want to practice? List a few habits that you would consider trying as a way to reach your aspirations. Remember to identify habits that are small, doable, and practical (realistic). Also favor habits that can be integrated into your existing daily routines.

Examples: Daily walk. Park my car farther away from my destination. Use the stairs every time there is an opportunity.

_____

_____

_____

_____

_____

_____

CREATE

Now, when you are set on what new habits you want to commit to, consider the context of your life and make sure you remove all reasons to say no and make it as easy as you can to say yes!

Example: I commit to walking 20 minutes every day before my first meal, together with my walking buddy.

What? _____

_____

When? _____

How? _____

_____

I commit to: _____

_____

_____

_____

_____

_____

_____

CELEBRATE

Be your own cheerleader! Every day you practice the habit, you will celebrate with a pat on the shoulder and say "Well done!"

RECIPES

CURED SALMON

Cured salmon, or gravlax, is a Swedish staple. Its versatility allows it to be used for a wide range of occasions. You cure it, slice it as is, and put it on a sandwich or make appetizers. This combination of sugar and salt acts as a curing agent, drawing out moisture from the fish and infusing it with a subtle sweetness and herbaceous aroma.

INGREDIENTS (MAKES ABOUT 20 SLICES)

- 1 ½ lb salmon: one fresh fillet with skin on
- 3 tbsp salt
- 1 ¾ tbsp sugar
- Freshly-ground pepper to taste (black or white)

HOW TO MAKE IT

1. Usually, when you buy salmon, it has been frozen; if not, make sure to do that.
2. Start by making a few cuts with a knife in the skin so the marinade can penetrate better.
3. Mix the sugar, salt, and crushed or ground pepper, and sprinkle it on both sides of the salmon fillet. Make sure to spread it out evenly.
4. You can then place the salmon fillet, with a plastic cover and some weight on top of it, in the refrigerator for 12–24 hours.

Now the cured salmon is ready to be sliced as thinly as you can without cutting into the skin. This takes some practice, but you will get the hang of it!

Tip: Try to buy a piece of quality fish that is evenly thick.

FRÖKNÄCKE

This recipe has become one of my staples over the past many years. There are many variations of this type of cracker. My version is flour-free, and if you have any allergies, you can, of course, adjust the ingredients to something else that works for you.

INGREDIENTS (MAKES TWO SHEETS OF FRÖKNÄCKE)

- 200 g of sunflower seeds
- ½ cup whole flaxseed
- ½ cup sesame seeds
- 1 cup pumpkin seeds
- 2 tbsp psyllium husk
- 2 tbsp almond flour
- 1 tsp salt
- 2 cups hot water
- ¼ cup poppy seeds
- salt flakes

HOW TO MAKE IT

1. Preheat the oven to 320°F.
2. Mix everything except the poppy seeds and sea salt in a bowl, and let the batter stand and swell for about 15 minutes.
3. Spread the batter thinly on two sheets lined with parchment paper.
4. Sprinkle with the poppy seeds and a little sea salt.
5. Bake for about 60–70 minutes.
6. Let the cracker sheets cool slightly, then loosen them carefully from the baking parchment. Store in a dry place.

Tip: Eat crackers with the sliced cured salmon.

FABRICE'S SOURDOUGH BREAD

I've been baking bread for as long as I can remember. A while back, I realized my friend Fabrice Braunrot was baking bread as well, and for the same reason: trying to get the healthiest bread without sacrificing taste. Below is the bread Fabrice came up with to reach his goal, which I'm making at home since he shared the recipe with me. You will need some active sourdough starter to make this.

"Avoiding insulin resistance has been a key part of my approach to wellness. Cutting sugar and processed carbohydrates from my diet has been central to that plan. That said I am a keen baker and huge lover of bread, pizza and English muffins. I discovered that I could 'have my bread and eat it' if I harnessed the age-old technique of natural fermentation using the beneficial microbes that literally float in the air around us. Enough people asked and I created fourthingsbread.com to get my bread to people who care about their metabolic well-being as much as they love a great slice of toast." —Fabrice Braunrot

---

FIRST THINGS FIRST: FEED YOUR STARTER

1. In a bowl, mix 4 oz of your starter with 4 oz of filtered water and 4 oz of flour.
2. Refrigerate for at least 24 hours before you use it.

> **Tip:** You can leave the starter out for an hour or so, to pick up some bacteria from the air, before you put it in the fridge.

INGREDIENTS (MAKES 1 LOAF)

- 18 oz flour
- 10 oz water
- 8 oz sourdough starter
- ½–1 tbsp salt

MAKING THE DOUGH

1. Take 8 oz of the starter when it is bubbly. Mix in 10 oz of filtered water plus 18 oz of flour plus ½–1 tbsp salt.
2. Knead it with your hands and make it into a ball. Put the dough in a bowl with a cover over it for about 48 hours.

TIME TO BAKE THE BREAD

1. The evening or morning before you are going to bake, take out the dough and knead it some (add slightly more flour if needed). Put it in a loaf pan and let it sit out on the counter to rise overnight or during the day. This is typically 12 or more hours.
2. When it has risen to the top of the loaf pan, cut into the dough lengthwise with a sharp knife.
3. Bake it in the oven at 350°F for 50–60 minutes, depending on your oven.
4. Remove to a cooling rack.

This bread I slice thin and eat toasted in the morning with butter, cheese, and cucumber, which my grandkids call "mormor's sandwich."

Tip: The cuts create openings through which moisture can escape during baking, resulting in a crisp and well-developed crust.

AYURVEDA SOUP
(ANTI-INFLAMMATORY)

A few years ago, my daughters and I tried to start a new tradition of going on "girls weekends," and this soup is from that wonderful time we had together. It is a constant reminder for me to make another trip happen with my girls.

INGREDIENTS (MAKES 4 SERVINGS)

- 1 small organic pumpkin, peeled, seeded, and cut into cubes
- 1 medium onion, finely chopped
- 1 tbsp of coconut oil
- 2 garlic cloves, minced
- 1½ tbsp minced, peeled fresh ginger
- 1 tsp ground cumin
- ¼ tsp ground cardamom
- ½ tsp coriander
- ¾ tsp red pepper flakes
- 1 cup coconut milk (unsweetened)
- 3 cups water
- 1½ tsp brown mustard seeds
- 1½ tsp Himalayan salt

HOW TO MAKE IT

1. Heat the oil in a heavy pot over medium heat. Add the onion and sauté until translucent for 3–4 minutes.
2. Add the garlic and ginger and sauté, stirring for another few minutes.
3. Add the cumin, coriander, cardamom, and red pepper flakes and stir.
4. Add the pumpkin, salt, coconut milk, and water; stir everything and simmer until the pumpkin is cooked thoroughly for about 40 minutes.
5. While the soup is cooking, place the mustard seeds in a small skillet over medium-high heat and cook until they pop, about 15 seconds.

6. Add the mustard seeds to the cooked soup.
7. Leave the soup on the stove to cool and for the flavors to mature for another 30–45 minutes. Transfer everything to a blender and puree until smooth.
8. Taste and adjust the flavor with salt.

GINGER SHOT

I've been enjoying hot water with lemon and/or ginger for as long as I can remember. This recipe is an option for that and has more of a kick to it. Try it if you are looking for a pick-me-up or feeling somewhat under the weather. The garlic and ginger make it amazing!

INGREDIENTS (MAKES 2 SERVINGS)

- 1 tbsp grated turmeric
- 1 tbsp grated ginger (peeled or not)
- ¼ tsp black pepper

- ½ lemon, cut fine
- 1 tsp crushed garlic
- Dash cayenne pepper (or more if you want it hot!)

HOW TO MAKE IT

1. Combine everything in a small container. I like to use mason jars with lids.
2. Mix until everything is well incorporated.
3. Save the paste in the refrigerator until you want to use it. When you want to use it, add 1 tsp of the immunity paste to warm or cold water.

An alternative is to mix it all with water in your high-speed mixer and drink it as is. It can sit in the refrigerator for a day or two like this.

PARTING WORDS

The fact that you've been reading this book suggests that you are not only open but also eager to figure out a better way to live a healthier life. I want to celebrate you for your commitment and willingness to explore new ideas—at least some of which probably seemed unusual or surprising at first.

While neither the scientific literature nor the plethora of media reports on how to live a healthier life are wrong or misdirected, I fear that they have contributed to the exhaustion and confusion many people feel when trying to figure out exactly what they should be doing. For those reasons, among others, I've used my own experiences to try to curate a set of daily habits that will go a long way toward helping most people improve their overall well-being.

> *My approach is one of holistic integration. Specialization is helpful in many ways, but we can often get lost in the details.*

Yes, I'm a dental professional as well as a public health advocate, but I'm also a wife, a mother, and a grandmother. And I use my own human experiences to describe and define the technical information I'm presenting in ways that I believe will speak to you more personally and directly than any study or textbook—although those, of course, provide the underpinnings for everything I have to say.

Because I can imagine that the idea of making so many changes in so many aspects of your life might seem a bit daunting right now, I want to share another of my own experiences—the process of writing this book. It felt intimidating at first because, after all, I'd never written a book before. But my purpose was clear, and I knew it was important, so I was willing to take the steps I knew were necessary to reach my goal. First, I had to commit to a weekly writing schedule. Accountability is an important first step when you're creating a new habit. At first, even an hour a day seemed too intimidating, so I settled on half an hour.

Once my schedule was in place, I asked myself an extremely important question: How can I make my writing practice enjoyable and enriching? Again—as I've told you—you're not going to keep doing something you don't want or like to do. One method I found was to walk while I was thinking about what I wanted to say. Walking helped me to clarify my thoughts, and it also helped make my commitment feel like less of a chore. If I felt stuck, I'd take myself on a walk and dictate my thoughts to my phone.

If you're ready to commit to starting to make at least some of the changes you've just read about, think of a plan to which you are ready and able to commit in order to accomplish what you want. Here are a few tips to get you started.

- Don't take on too much all at once. By doing that you may soon be overwhelmed and quit before you ever get there. Remember, life is like a long and complicated math problem; it takes more than one step to get to the right answer.

- You can take on a couple of new changes as long as they are moving you toward your destination.

- "Change" is an action verb. Unfortunately, you can't just contemplate changing and make it magically happen. If that were so, we'd all be losing weight and getting fit just by thinking about it.

- Try to surround yourself with people who inspire and support you.

- Be focused but flexible. Over time, for any number of reasons, including the progress you've made, you may need to tweak your plan to be sure it is still the best one for you. Being open to change can also be a habit. Say "yes" to any opportunities to advance your goals.

The suggestions I've given you along the way in this book are not quick fixes, but I believe that once you begin to implement them, you'll notice a positive difference in your life and your health fairly quickly. Take one step at a time!

Undertaking long-term change can be challenging, but keeping the end in mind will keep you motivated, and the end will more than justify the means. Simply knowing how you want to live your life and what makes you happy, and slowly but surely moving toward your goals, is my definition of success. In fact, I believe that you are most successful when you continue to learn and to grow. If it helps, think of yourself as a professional athlete who is constantly training and improving to be the best you can be.

Personally, I'm excited to learn more about dental and overall health from future research, and my hope for you is that you, too, will continue moving forward on your own path to doing the same.

REFERENCES

CHAPTER 1: OPEN WIDE

"The common risk factor approach: a rational basis for promoting oral health," Sheiham, A., & Watt, R. G. (2000), https://pubmed.ncbi.nlm.nih.gov/11106011/

Oral Homeostatis/Oral Microbiome
"The Importance of Homeostasis in Oral and Systemic Health," Abner Escobedo, https://www.alliedacademies.org/articles/the-importance-of-homeostasis-in-oral-and-systemic-health.pdf, Journal of Oral Medicine and Surgery 3(1), 2020

"Defining the oral microbiome by whole-genome sequencing and resistome analysis: the complexity of the healthy picture," Caselli, E., Fabbri, C., D'Accolti, M. et al. BMC Microbiol 20, 120 (2020), https://doi.org/10.1186/s12866-020-01801-y

"Oral Microbiome and Health," Sharma N, Bhatia S, Sodhi AS, Batra N. AIMS Microbiol. 2018 Jan 12;4(1):42-66. doi: 10.3934/microbiol.2018.1.42. PMID: 31294203; PMCID: PMC6605021

"Physiological properties of Streptococcus mutans UA159 biofilm-detached cells," Jia Liu, Jun-Qi Ling, Kai Zhang, Christine D Wu, FEMS Microbiol Lett. 2013 Mar; 340(1):11-8. doi: 10.1111/1574-6968.12066. Epub 2013 Jan 14. PMID: 23278289

"The oral microbiome and human health," Yoshihisa Yamashita, Toru Takeshita, J Oral Sci. 2017;59(2):201-206. doi: 10.2334/josnusd.16-0856. PMID: 28637979

"Oral microbiome: Unveiling the fundamentals," Priya Nimish Deo and Revati Deshmukh, J Oral Maxillofac Pathol. 2019 Jan-Apr;23(1):122-128. doi: 10.4103/jomfp.JOMFP_304_18. PMID: 31110428; PMCID: PMC6503789

"Assessment of salivary calcium, phosphate, magnesium, pH, and flow rate in healthy subjects, periodontitis, and dental caries," K. S. Rajesh, Zareena, Shashikanth Hegde, and M. S. Arun Kumar, Contemp Clin Dent. 2015 Oct-Dec;6(4):461-5. doi: 10.4103/0976-237X.169846. PMID: 26681848; PMCID: PMC4678541

"Oral microbiota: A new view of body health," Maoyang Lu, Songyu Xuan, Zhao Wang, https://www.sciencedirect.com/science/article/pii/S2213453018301642?via%3Dihub, https://doi.org/10.1016/j.fshw.2018.12.001

The Stephan Curve
"The Stephan Curve revisited," William H Bowen, https://pubmed.ncbi.nlm.nih.gov/23224410/, Bowen WH. The Stephan Curve revisited. Odontology. 2013 Jan; 101(1):2-8. doi: 10.1007/s10266-012-0092-z. Epub 2012 Dec 6. PMID: 23224410

Gum Disease
"Periodontal (gum) disease," WHO Oral health, https://www.who.int/news-room/fact-sheets/detail/oral-health

"Facts About Adult Oral Health," CDC, https://www.cdc.gov/oralhealth/basics/adult-oral-health/

"Problem in the gum," Bui FQ, Almeida-da-Silva CLC, Huynh B, Trinh A, Liu J, Woodward J, Asadi H, Ojcius DM, Biomed J. 2019 Feb;42(1):27-35. doi: 10.1016/j. bj.2018.12.001. Epub 2019 Mar 2. PMID: 30987702; PMCID: PMC6468093

Books

Mouth Health Come Clean, Ellie Phillips DDS, River Grove Books, 2018

Heal Your Oral Microbiome, Cass Nelson-Dooley, Ulysses Press, 2019

Happy Gut, Vincent Pedre, William Morrow, 2015

Eat, Sleep, Breathe Oral Health, Yasmin Chebbi, Independently published, 2020

Podcasts/YouTube

"Oral Microbiome—What it is and why it's important," Cass Nelson-Dooley, https://www.youtube.com/watch?v=vCAcWqQGpes

"What Really Causes Cavities?," https://www.youtube.com/

CHAPTER 2: THE BODY CONNECTION

WHO, https://www.who.int/news/item/18-11-2022-who-highlights-oral-health-neglect-affecting-nearly-half-of-the-world-s-population

"Systemic Diseases Caused by Oral Infection", Xiaojing Li, Kristin M. Kolltveit, Leif Tronstad, and Ingar Olsen, Clin Microbiol Rev. 2000 Oct;13(4):547-58. doi: 10.1128/CMR.13.4.547. PMID: 11023956; PMCID: PMC88948

"Association between periodontal pathogens and systemic disease," Fiona Q Bui, Cassio Luiz Coutinho Almeida-da-Silva, Brandon Huynh, Alston Trinh, Jessica Liu, Jacob Woodward, Homer Asadi, David M Ojcius, Biomed J. 2019 Feb;42(1):27-35. doi: 10.1016/j.bj.2018.12.001. Epub 2019 Mar 2. PMID: 30987702; PMCID: PMC6468093

"Periodontal disease and systemic conditions: a bidirectional relationship," Kim J, Amar S. Periodontal disease and systemic conditions: a bidirectional relationship. Odontology. 2006 Sep;94(1):10-21. doi: 10.1007/s10266-006-0060-6. PMID: 16998613; PMCID: PMC2443711

"Traditional Chinese medicine tongue inspection: an examination of the inter- and intrapractitioner reliability for specific tongue characteristics," Minah Kim, Deirdre Cobbin, Christopher Zaslawski, https://pubmed.ncbi.nlm.nih.gov/18564955/

"Oral health and atherosclerotic cardiovascular disease: A review," Gianos E, Jackson EA, Tejpal A, Aspry K, O'Keefe J, Aggarwal M, Jain A, Itchhaporia D, Williams K, Batts T, Allen KE, Yarber C, Ostfeld RJ, Miller M, Reddy K, Freeman AM, Fleisher KE. Am J Prev Cardiol. 2021 Apr 5;7:100179. doi: 10.1016/j.ajpc.2021.100179. PMID: 34611631; PMCID: PMC8387275

"Association between periodontal pathogens and systemic disease," Fiona Q Bui, Cassio Luiz Coutinho Almeida-da-Silva, Brandon Huynh, Alston Trinh, Jessica Liu, Jacob Woodward, Homer Asadi, David M Ojcius, Biomed J. 2019 Feb;42(1):27-35. doi: 10.1016/j.bj.2018.12.001. Epub 2019 Mar 2. PMID: 30987702; PMCID: PMC6468093

Diabetes

"Gingival inflammatory infiltrate analysis in patients with chronic periodontitis and diabetes mellitus," Olteanu M, Surlin P, Oprea B, Rauten AM, Popescu RM, Ni_u M, Camen GC, Caraivan O. Rom J Morphol Embryol. 2011;52(4):1311-7. PMID: 22203939

"Association between periodontal pathogens and systemic disease," Bui, Fiona Q., Cássio Luiz Coutinho Almeida-da-Silva, Brandon Huynh, Alston Trinh, Jessica Liu, Jacob Woodward, Homer Asadi and David M. Ojcius, https://www.sciencedirect.com/science/article/pii/S2319417018302634

"Diabetes, Gum Disease, & Other Dental Problems," NIH, https://www.niddk.nih.gov/health-information/diabetes/overview/preventing-problems/gum-disease-dental-problems, CDC, https://www.cdc.gov/diabetes/managing/diabetes-oral-health.html

"What Is Diabetes?," NIH, https://www.niddk.nih.gov/health-information/diabetes/overview/what-is-diabetes

"Type-2 Diabetes," Centers for Disease Control and Prevention, https://www.cdc.gov/diabetes/basics/type2.html

Alzheimer's Disease

"Tooth loss in older adults linked to higher risk of dementia," National Inst of Aging, https://www.nia.nih.gov/news/tooth-loss-older-adults-linked-higher-risk-dementia

"Clinical and Bacterial Markers of Periodontitis and Their Association with Incident All-Cause and Alzheimer's Disease Dementia in a Large National Survey," May A Beydoun, Hind A Beydoun, Sharmin Hossain, Ziad W El-Hajj, Jordan Weiss, Alan B Zonderman, J Alzheimer's Dis. 2020;75(1):157-172. doi: 10.3233/JAD-200064. PMID: 32280099.

Colorectal Cancer

"Oral health and risk of colorectal cancer: results from three cohort studies and a meta-analysis," Harvard and other in Boston mostly, https://www.sciencedirect.com/science/article/pii/S0923753419356972

"Oral Health and Colorectal Cancer Risk? In a study, researchers found an association between periodontal disease, tooth loss, and conditions associated with colorectal cancer.," Am. Assoc For Cancer Research, https://www.aacr.org/patients-caregivers/progress-against-cancer/oral-health-and-colorectal-cancer-risk/

"Gum disease associated with higher gastrointestinal, colon cancer risk," Harvard School of Public Health, https://www.hsph.harvard.edu/news/hsph-in-the-news/gum-disease-gastrointestinal-cancer-risk/

Respiratory Disease

"Oral health and respiratory infection," Philippe Mojon, J Can Dent Assoc. 2002 Jun;68(6):340-5. PMID: 12034069.

"Respiratory disease and the role of oral bacteria," Isaac S. Gomes-Filho, Johelle S. Passos and Simone Seixas da Cruz, J Oral Microbiol. 2010 Dec 21;2. doi: 10.3402/jom.v2i0.5811. PMID: 21523216; PMCID: PMC3084574.

Adverse Pregnancy Outcomes

"Pregnancy and Oral Health," CDC, https://www.cdc.gov/oralhealth/publications/features/pregnancy-and-oral-health.html

"Oral Health in Pregnancy," Erin Hartnett, Judith Haber, Barbara Krainovich-Miller, Abigail Bella, Anna Vasilyeva, https://www.sciencedirect.com/science/article/pii/S0884217516301599

"Oral care in pregnancy," Zeynep Yenen and Tijen Ataça, J Turk Ger Gynecol Assoc. 2019 Nov 28;20(4):264-268. doi: 10.4274/jtgga.galenos.2018.2018.0139. Epub 2018 Dec 17. PMID: 30556662; PMCID: PMC6883753

"Bleeding gums in pregnancy," NHS source, https://www.nhs.uk/pregnancy/related-conditions/common-symptoms/bleeding-gums

Autoimmune Conditions
"Leaky gut: What is it, and what does it mean for you?," Marcelo Campos, MD, Contributor Harvard, https://www.health.harvard.edu/blog/leaky-gut-what-is-it-and-what-does-it-mean-for-you-2017092212451

"The microbiome of the oral mucosa in irritable bowel syndrome," Nicolaas H. Fourie, Dan Wang, Sarah K. Abey, LeeAnne B. Sherwin, Paule V. Joseph, Bridgett Rahim-Williams, Eric G. Ferguson, and Wendy A. Henderson, Gut Microbes. 2016 Jul 3;7(4):286-301. doi: 10.1080/19490976.2016.1162363. Epub 2016 Mar 10. PMID: 26963804; PMCID: PMC4988452

"Periodontal disease and rheumatoid arthritis: the evidence accumulates for complex pathobiologic interactions," Clifton O. Bingham and Malini Monib, Curr Opin Rheumatol. 2013 May;25(3):345-53. doi: 10.1097/BOR.0b013e32835fb8ec. PMID: 23455329; PMCID: PMC4495574

"Association between periodontal pathogens and systemic disease," Fiona Bui, https://www.sciencedirect.com/science/article/pii/S2319417018302634

"Everything You Need to Know About Acid Reflux and GERD," Medically reviewed by Youssef (Joe) Soliman, MD— By Jessica DiGiacinto — Updated on Oct 20, 2021, https://www.healthline.com/health/gerd

"Oral Health Celiac Disease Tooth Development and Soft Tissue Defects," Ted Malahias, DDS, https://celiac.org/about-celiac-disease/related-conditions/oral-health/

"Sjogren's Disease," NIH, https://www.niams.nih.gov/health-topics/sjogrens-syndrome

Red Swollen Tongue
"Oral manifestations in vitamin B12 deficiency patients with or without history of gastrectomy," Jihoon Kim, Moon-Jong Kim, and Hong-Seop Kho, https://www.ncbi.nlm.nih.gov/pmc/articles/PMC4884371/

"Everything You Need to Know About Tongue Swelling," Medically reviewed by Elaine K. Luo, M.D. — By Darla Burke, https://www.healthline.com/health/tongue-problems#causes

Candida
"Candida infections of the mouth, throat, and esophagus," CDC, https://www.cdc.gov/fungal/diseases/candidiasis/thrush/index.html

Mouth Sores
"Aphthous Stomatitis," Michael C. Plewa; Kingshuk Chatterjee 2022, https://www.ncbi.nlm.nih.gov/books/NBK431059/

"Mouth Sores: Symptoms, Treatment, and Prevention Methods," Avi Varma, MD, MPH, AAHIVS, FAAFP, By Julie Roddickand Heather Hobb, https://www.healthline.com/health/mouth-sores

"Oral Lichen Planus," Last reviewed by a Cleveland Clinic medical professional on 07/25/2022., https://my.clevelandclinic.org/health/diseases/17875-oral-lichen-planus

Burning Mouth Syndrome
"Burning Mouth Syndrome," Last reviewed by a Cleveland Clinic medical professional on 06/26/2022., https://my.clevelandclinic.org/health/diseases/14463-burning-mouth-syndrome

"Burning Mouth Syndrome," R. Aravindhan, Santhanam Vidyalakshmi, Muniapillai Siva Kumar, Satheesh, Murali Balasubramanium, Srinivas Prasad, https://www.ncbi.nlm.nih.gov/pmc/articles/PMC4157273/

"Burning Mouth Syndrome," Gregory P. Bookout; Megan Ladd; Radley E. Short., https://www.ncbi.nlm.nih.gov/books/NBK519529/

Books
Whole-Body Dentistry, Mark A Breiner, https://wholebodymed.com/staff/dr-mark-breiner-dds/

Mouth-Body Connection, Gerald Curatola, https://www.rejuvdentist.com/meet-dr-gerry-curatola-new-york-ny/

Eat Sleep Move Breathe: The Beginner's Guide to Living A Healthy Lifestyle, Lars Thestrup, Jennifer Pfleghaar, Connor Martin, Kharis Publishing, an imprint of Kharis Media LLC, 2020

Eat Sleep Breathe Oral Health, Yasmin N Chebbi, Independently published, 2020

The Dental Diet, Steven Lin, Hay House Inc, 2018

GUT, Giulia Enders, Greystone Books, 2015

Happy Gut, Vincent Pedre, William Morrow, 2015, Vincent Pedre website, https://pedremd.com/

Podcasts/YouTube
"Teeth: Your body's early warning system" TEDxSaltLakeCity, Marielle Pariseau DMD, https://youtu.be/YXSgL-aYlwg?si=jF6drC96S1fwM2JC

"Your Gut Microbiome: The Most Important Organ You've Never Heard Of" | TEDxFargo, Erika Ebbel Angle, https://www.youtube.com/watch?v=B9RruLkAUm8

CHAPTER 3: HABITS: WHAT THEY ARE, WHAT THEY DO, AND HOW TO MAKE NEW ONES

"Pavlov's Dogs Experiment and Pavlovian Conditioning Response," Saul Mcleod, PhD, https://www.simplypsychology.org/pavlov.html

The Power of Habit: Why We Do What We Do in Life and Business, Charles Duhigg, Random House, 2014

"There's a SMART Way to Write Management's Goals and Objectives" George Doran, https://www.scirp.org/(S(czeh2tfqyw2orz553k1w0r45))/reference/ReferencesPapers.aspx?ReferenceID=1459599

Tiny Habits: The Small Changes That Change Everything, BJ Fogg, Harvest, 2020

"Habits—A Repeat Performance" full article as PDF, David T. Neal, Wendy Wood, and Jeffrey M. Quinn, https://dornsife.usc.edu/assets/sites/545/docs/Wendy_Wood_Research_Articles/Habits/Neal.Wood.Quinn.2006_Habits_a_repeat_performance.pdf

"Making health habitual: the psychology of 'habit-formation' and general practice," Benjamin Gardner, Phillippa Lally, Jane Wardle, https://www.ncbi.nlm.nih.gov/pmc/articles/PMC3505409/

Books
No Chance Encounter, Kaj Pollak, Findhorn Pr, 1997. No Chance Encounter is a short, sharp, ingenious course in how to transform our own lives and the lives of those around us through the way we handle our daily encounters with others.

Hello Habits: A Minimalist's Guide to a Better Life, Fumio Sasaki, W. W. Norton & Company, 2021

Atomic Habits, James Clear, Avery, 2018

Good Habits, Bad Habits, Wendy Wood, Farrar, Straus and Giroux, 2019

Small Move, Big Change, Caroline L. Arnold, Penguin Books; Reprint edition, 2014

Podcasts/YouTube
"Atomic Habits: How to Get 1% Better Every Day," James Clear, https://www.youtube.com/watch?v=U_nzqnXWvSo

"The 3 life-changing ideas in James Clear's Atomic Habits," Thomas Frank, https://www.youtube.com/watch?v=sJwZLTztg5s

"Tiny Habits: Core Message," Productivity Game, https://www.youtube.com/watch?v=S_8e-6ZHKLs

"Tiny Habits: Small Changes Change Everything with BJ Fogg," Brilliant Miller, https://www.youtube.com/watch?v=uTawbZA7odY

"Forget big change, start with a tiny habit: BJ Fogg at TEDxFremont," BJ Fogg, https://www.youtube.com/watch?v=AdKUJxjn-R8

CHAPTER 4: HOW, WHEN, WHAT TO EAT

Eating Habits
"Health and Economic Costs of Chronic Diseases," CDC, https://www.cdc.gov/chronicdisease/about/costs/

"Let food be thy medicine . . .", BMJ 2004; 328, https://doi.org/10.1136/bmj.328.7433.0-g

"Nutrition and Physical Degeneration", Weston Price, Price-Pottenger Nutrition Foundation, 2009

"The Lost American Diet," Dan Buettner, https://www.youtube.com/watch?v=pMNQflEDaWg

"The Swedish Fika Ritual," Tor Kjolberg, https://www.dailyscandinavian.com/the-swedish-fika-ritual/

Intermittent Fasting
"Intermittent Fasting," Cynthia Thurlow, https://youtu.be/A6Dkt7zylmk

"Circadian rhythm and intermittent fasting," Satchin Panda, https://youtu.be/fciGNBN0nKM

"The COMPLETE Beginners Guide To Intermittent Fasting For LONGEVITY," Interview on Dr Chatterjee podcast with Dr Jason Funge, https://youtu.be/IXsKwQxhwjs

"The Big IF Study—Intermittent fasting ZOE nutrition and science," ZOE Health Study, https://health-study.joinzoe.com/intermittent-fasting

Chewing
"Jaws: The Story of a Hidden Epidemic," Dr Ron Ehrlich interviews Sandra Kahn, https://www.youtube.com/watch?v=GTZOi2KXU04

Breath, James Nestor, Riverhead Books, 2020

The Story of the Human Body: Evolution, Health, and Disease, Daniel Lieberman, Vintage, 2013

Food Rules: An Eater's Manual, Michael Pollan, Penguin Books, 2021

In The Defense of Food, Michael Pollan, Penguin Books, 2008

"Physiology, Glucose Metabolism," Mihir N. Nakrani; Robert H. Wineland; Fatima Anjum, StatPearls Publishing; 2023 https://www.ncbi.nlm.nih.gov/books/NBK560599/

Sugar
"The Sugar Conspiracy," Ian Leslie, https://www.theguardian.com/society/2016/apr/07/the-sugar-conspiracy-robert-lustig-john-yudkin

Pure, White and Deadly, John Yudkin, Penguin Books, 2013

Seven Countries Study, Dr Ancel Keys, https://www.sevencountriesstudy.com/

"A systematic comparison of sugar content in low-fat vs regular versions of food," P. K. Nguyen, S. Lin, and P Heidenreich, https://www.ncbi.nlm.nih.gov/pmc/articles/PMC4742721/

"Fructose, insulin resistance, and metabolic dyslipidemia," Heather Basciano, Lisa Federico, Khosrow Adeli, https://pubmed.ncbi.nlm.nih.gov/15723702/

"Just eaten and you're hungry again? How big dips in blood sugar levels make you eat more and can ruin your diet," Anthea Rowan, https://www.scmp.com/lifestyle/health-wellness/article/3135492/just-eaten-and-youre-hungry-again-how-big-dips-blood

"The negative impact of sugarsweetened beverages on children's health: an update of the literature," Sara N. Bleich & Kelsey A. Vercammen, https://bmcobes.biomedcentral.com/articles/10.1186/s40608-017-0178-9

Omega 3 and 6
"The importance of the ratio of omega-6/omega-3 essential fatty acids," A.P Simopoulos, https://doi.org/10.1016/S0753-3322(02)00253-6

"Omega 3 vs Omega 6: How Do They Compare?," Dr. Venn-Watson, November 11, 2020, https://fatty15.com/blogs/news/what-is-the-difference-between-omega-3-and-omega-6

"Omega-6 vegetable oils as a driver of coronary heart disease: the oxidized linoleic acid hypothesis," James J DiNicolantonio and James H O'Keefe, https://www.ncbi.nlm.nih.gov/pmc/articles/PMC6196963/

"Does cooking with vegetable oils increase the risk of chronic diseases?: a systematic review," Carmen Sayon-Orea, Silvia Carlos, Miguel A Martínez-Gonzalez, https://www.cambridge.org/core/services/aop-cambridge-core/content/view/AF44097B0E9C4FF9BD44F1D55CD353D6/S0007114514002931a.pdf/div-class-title-does-cooking-with-vegetable-oils-increase-the-risk-of-chronic-diseases-a-systematic-review-div.pdf

The Nutrition Source HARVARD, https://www.hsph.harvard.edu/nutritionsource/what-should-you-eat/protein/

"How to Optimize Your Omega-6 to Omega-3 Ratio," Medically reviewed by Kim Chin, RD, Nutrition By Kris Gunnars, BSc Updated on Feb 15, 2023, https://www.healthline.com/nutrition/optimize-omega-6-omega-3-ratio

"The 3 Most Important Types of Omega-3 Fatty Acids," Freydis Hjalmarsdottir, MS, https://www.healthline.com/nutrition/3-types-of-omega-3

Better Fats
Good Fat, Bad Fat, Romy Dollé, Primal Nutrition, Inc., 2016

"Water, Hydration and Health," Barry M. Popkin, Kristen E. D'Anci, and Irwin H. Rosenberg, https://www.ncbi.nlm.nih.gov/pmc/articles/PMC2908954/

Why We Get Fat, Gary Taubes, Knopf, 2010

Protein
"Protein Intake and Oral Health in Older Adults—A Narrative Review," Thilini N. Jayasinghe, Sanaa Harrass, Sharon Erdrich, Shalinie King, and Joerg Eberhard, https://www.ncbi.nlm.nih.gov/pmc/articles/PMC9653899/

The Nutrition Source, Harvard School of Public Health, https://www.hsph.harvard.edu/nutritionsource/what-should-you-eat/protein/

"Dietary protein: an essential nutrient for bone health," Jean-Phillippe Bonjour, https://pubmed.ncbi.nlm.nih.gov/16373952/

"Dietary protein to maximize resistance training: a review and examination of protein spread and change theories," John D. Bosse and Brian M. Dixon, https://pubmed.ncbi.nlm.nih.gov/22958314/

"The Effects of High Protein Diets on Thermogenesis, Satiety and Weight Loss: A Critical Review," Thomas L. Halton and Frank B. Hu, https://pubmed.ncbi.nlm.nih.gov/15466943/

"10 Science-Backed Reasons to Eat More Protein," Kris Gunnars, BSc—Updated on Mar 8, 2019, https://www.healthline.com/nutrition/10-reasons-to-eat-more-protein

"Protein Intake and Oral Health in Older Adults," Scholarly Community Encyclopedia, https://encyclopedia.pub/entry/35883

"Effect of a high-protein breakfast on the postprandial ghrelin response, Wendy A. M. Blom, Anne Lluch, Annette Stafleu, Sophie Vinoy, Jens J Holst, Gertjan Schaafsma, Henk F. J. Hendriks, https://pubmed.ncbi.nlm.nih.gov/16469977/

Calcium
"Hypercalcemia: What Happens If You Have Too Much Calcium?," HEALTHLINE Medically reviewed by Judith Marcin, M.D., https://www.healthline.com/health/hypercalcemia

Vitamin D
"Vitamin D Deficiency and Oral Health: A Comprehensive Review," João Botelho, Vanessa Machado, Luís Proença, Ana Sintra Delgado, and José João Mendes, https://www.ncbi.nlm.nih.gov/pmc/articles/PMC7285165/

The Dental Diet, Steven Lin, Hay House Inc., 2018

Vitamin C
"Beneficial Effects of Vitamin C in Maintaining Optimal Oral Health," Julienne Murererehe, Anne Marie Uwitonze, Pacifique Nikuze, Jay Patel, and Mohammed S. Razzaque, https://www.ncbi.nlm.nih.gov/pmc/articles/PMC8784414/

Vitamin K
"Vitamin K Metabolism," Paul Newman & Martin J. Shearer, https://link.springer.com/chapter/10.1007/978-1-4899-1789-8_19

"How Vitamin K2 Fuels Jaw Growth," Steven Lin website, https://www.drstevenlin.com/vitamin-k2-deficiency-effects/

"Proper Calcium Use: Vitamin K2 as a Promoter of Bone and Cardiovascular Health," Katarzyna Maresz, PhD, https://www.ncbi.nlm.nih.gov/pmc/articles/PMC4566462/pdf/34-39.pdf

Vitamin E
"The effect of Vitamin E supplementation on treatment of chronic periodontitis," Parichehr Behfarnia, Mina Dadmehr, Seyedeh Negin Hosseini, and Seyed Amir Mirghaderi, https://www.ncbi.nlm.nih.gov/pmc/articles/PMC8428286/

General
Nutrition and Human Oral Health, Kirstin Vach and Johan Peter Woelber Eds, https://www.mdpi.com/books/book/5728-nutrition-and-human-oral-health

"Nutrition and Physical Degeneration: A Comparison of Primitive and Modern Diets and Their Effects," C. F. Elzea, published 1939, https://www.semanticscholar.org/paper/Nutrition-and-Physical-Degeneration%3A-A-Comparison-Elzea/eb03439a9543410a8a45d24d3b82de7e6b9e3d67

"12 Graphs That Show Why People Get Fat," Kris Gunnars, Authority Nutrition Sep 4, 2014, https://www.businessinsider.com/12-graphs-that-show-why-people-get-fat-2014-9

"United States Dietary Trends Since 1800: Lack of Association Between Saturated Fatty Acid Consumption and Non-communicable Diseases," Joyce H. Lee, Miranda Duster, Timothy Roberts, and Orrin Devinsky, https://www.frontiersin.org/articles/10.3389/fnut.2021.748847/full#h1

"Sugar and Dental Caries," WHO, November 2017, https://www.who.int/news-room/fact-sheets/detail/sugars-and-dental-caries

Books

The Dental Diet, Steven Lin, Hay House Inc., 2018

Eat Dirt, Dr. Josh Axe, DC, DNM, CNS, Macmillan, 2016

The Art of Gathering: How We Meet and Why It Matters, Priya Parker, Riverhead Books, 2018

The Pegan Diet, Dr Mark Hyman, Little, Brown Spark, 2021

Food Fix, Dr. Mark Hyman, Little, Brown Spark, 2020

Eat Fat Get Thin, Dr Mark Hyman, Little, Brown Spark, 2016

The Big Fat Surprise, Nina Teicholz, Simon & Schuster, 2014

Vitamin K2 and the Calcium Paradox, Kate Rheaume-Bleue, Harper, 2013

Effortless Healing, Joseph Mercola, Harmony, 2015

Nutrition and Physical Degeneration, Weston Price DDS, Price-Pottenger Nutrition Foundation, 2009

Spoon Fed, Tim Spector, Vintage, 2022

The Mouth-Body Connection: a 28-Day Program to Create a Healthy Mouth, Reduce Inflammation, and Prevent Disease throughout the Body, Dr. Gerry Curatola with Diane Reverand, Center Street, 2017

Podcasts/YouTube

"The Importance of Dental Care in Whole Body Health," Steven Lin at Broken Brain Podcast, https://podcasts.apple.com/us/podcast/15-the-importance-of-dental-care-in-whole-body-health/id1381257272?i=1000417544828

"How to Treat Cavities and Reverse Tooth Decay Naturally," Dr. Josh Axe, DC, DNM, CNS, https://www.youtube.com/watch?v=P6PZw52_1ig

"How to reverse Cavities Naturally," Dr. Josh Axe, DC, DNM, CNS, https://draxe.com/health/naturally-reverse-cavities-heal-tooth-decay/

"Clean Mouth, Clean Brain," Dr. Hyman Podcast, https://drhyman.com/blog/2019/12/03/clean-mouth-clean-brain/

"Sugar: The bitter Truth," Robert Lustig, https://youtu.be/dBnniua6-oM

"The Elephant in the kitchen," Robert Lustig, https://youtu.be/gmC4Rm5cpOl

"The Secrets of Sugar – the fifth estate," Robert Lustig, https://youtu.be/K3ksKkCOgTw

"The Latest Science on Gut Health (and How To Find The Right Diet For You)," Tim Spector interviewed by R Chatterjee, https://drchatterjee.com/tim-spector-the-latest-science-on-gut-health-and-how-to-find-the-right-diet-for-you/

"How to prevent cavities using an ancestral diet,"Steven Lin interviewed by Dhru Purohit, https://podcasts.apple.com/us/podcast/172-how-to-prevent-cavities-using-an-ancestral-diet/id1381257272?i=1000500799646

"Eating ourselves to death," Dr Casey Means interviewed by Bari Weiss, Honestly with Bari Weiss, https://www.levelshealth.com/podcasts/eating-ourselves-to-death-dr-casey-means

"Best foods for healthy teeth," Steven Lin, https://youtu.be/vzEHb-t0rm4

"Teeth: Your body's early warning system | Marielle Pariseau DMD | TEDxSaltLakeCity," Marielle Pariseau DMD, https://www.youtube.com/watch?v=YXSgL-aYlwg

"Sugar: Hiding in Plain Sight," Robert Lustig, https://www.ted.com/talks/robert_lustig_sugar_hiding_in_plain_sight

"Circadian theory of life," Sachin Panda, https://youtu.be/LJ9Ae_j_kJl

Websites
Gary Taubes website, https://garytaubes.com/works/

Blue Zones, https://www.bluezones.com/

CHAPTER 5: THE TRUTH ABOUT SLEEP

Sleeping Habits
Why We Sleep – Unlock the power of sleep and dreams, Matthew Walker PhD, Scribner, 2018

"Sleep is one of the most important but least understood aspects of our life, wellness, and longevity," Matthew Walker, M Walker on Dr Chatterjee Feel better Live More podcast #26 - https://podcasts.apple.com/ie/podcast/26-why-we-sleep-with-matthew-walker-part-1/id1333552422?i=1000415615744

"Interview about her book: The Sleep Revolution," Arianna Huffington at Google 2014, https://www.youtube.com/watch?v=jtagD45fCMo

Circadian Rhythm
"How to make your body clock work for you," Russell Foster from Oxford University interviewed on ZOE Science & Nutrition Podcast, https://youtu.be/E9Gt97G9qS8

Ghrelin and Leptin
"How To Sleep Better For Good Health: Matthew Walker | Bitesize," Dr Rangan Chatterjee interview MDr Matthew Walker, https://www.youtube.com/watch?v=QSU4CbYknqc&t=249s

Sleep Deprivation
"What Are Sleep Deprivation and Deficiency?," https://www.nhlbi.nih.gov/health/sleep-deprivation

"The impact of sleep deprivation on food desire in the human brain," Stephanie M. Greer, Andrea N. Goldstein, and Matthew P. Walker, https://www.ncbi.nlm.nih.gov/pmc/articles/PMC3763921/

"The connection between insomnia and dental problems," American Academy of Medical Orthodontics, https://medicalorthodontics.org/dental_articles/the-connection-between-insomnia-and-dental-problems/

"How to succeed? Get more sleep, Arianna Huffington at TED Women 2010," https://www.ted.com/talks/arianna_huffington_how_to_succeed_get_more_sleep

Sleep Apnea, Snoring, Bruxism

"Snoring and Sleep," Kent Smith, Dentist, Sleep Apnea Expert writer: Eric Suni, https://www.sleepfoundation.org/snoring

"Association between quality of sleep and chronic periodontitis: A case–control study in Malaysian population," Vijendra Pal Singh, Joe Yin Gan, Wei Ling Liew, Htoo Htoo Kyaw Soe, https://www.ncbi.nlm.nih.gov/pmc/articles/PMC6340225/

"TMJ Disorder Overview," Mayo Clinic, https://www.mayoclinic.org/diseases-conditions/tmj/symptoms-causes/syc-20350941

"The Link between Sleep Bruxism, Sleep Disordered Breathing and Temporomandibular Disorders: An Evidence-based Review," Ramesh Balasubramaniam, BDSc, MS; Gary D. Klasser, DMD; Peter A. Cistulli, MD, PhD; Gilles J. Lavigne, DDS, PhD, https://aadsm.org/docs/JDSM.1.1.27.pdf

"Tongue Function: An Underrecognized Component in the Treatment of Obstructive Sleep Apnea with Mandibular Repositioning Appliance," Wei Wang, Changping Di, Skaff Mona, Lin Wang, and Mark Hans, https://www.ncbi.nlm.nih.gov/pmc/articles/PMC6247694/

"Estimation of the global prevalence and burden of obstructive sleep apnoea: a literature-based analysis," Adam V Benjafield, PhD, Najib T Ayas, MD, https://www.thelancet.com/journals/lanres/article/PIIS2213-2600(19)30198-5/fulltext

"Evaluation of Sleep Habits and Disturbances Among US Adults, 2017–2020," Hongkun Di, MD; Yanjun Guo, MD, PhD; Iyas Daghlas, MD; et al, https://jamanetwork.com/journals/jamanetworkopen/fullarticle/2798209

"The Relationship between Sleep Bruxism and Obstructive Sleep Apnea Based on Polysomnographic Findings," Helena Martynowicz, Pawel Gac, Anna Brzecka, Rafal Poreba, Anna Wojakowska, Grzegorz Mazur, Joanna Smardz and Mieszko Wieckiewicz, https://www.ncbi.nlm.nih.gov/pmc/articles/PMC6832407/pdf/jcm-08-01653.pdf

"What is Sleep Apnea?," NIH national heart lung and blood institute, https://www.nhlbi.nih.gov/health/sleep-apnea

"Sleep apnoea is a common occurrence in females," Karl A. Franklin; Carin Sahlin; Hans Stenlund; and Eva Lindberg, https://erj.ersjournals.com/content/erj/41/3/610.full.pdf

"Is There a Connection Between Sleep Apnea and Teeth Grinding?," Eric Suni and John DeBanto Internal Medicine Physician, https://www.sleepfoundation.org/sleep-apnea/link-between-sleep-apnea-and-teeth-grinding

"Snoring and Sleep: A closer look at what snoring is as well as its causes, consequences, and treatments," Eric Suni, Kent Smith, https://www.sleepfoundation.org/snoring

"Obstructive Sleep Apnea in Women: Specific Issues and Interventions," Alison Wimms; Holger Woehrle; Sahisha Ketheeswaran; Dinesh Ramanan; and Jeffery Armitstead, https://www.ncbi.nlm.nih.gov/pmc/articles/PMC5028797/

"The Possible Connection Between Sleep Apnea and Teeth Grinding," Martinique Edwards, https://www.sleepapnea.org/sleep-health/teeth-grinding-and-sleep-apnea/

"The Relationship between Sleep Bruxism and Obstructive Sleep Apnea Based on Polysomnographic Findings," Helena Martynowicz; Pawel Gac; Anna Brzecka; Rafal Poreba; Anna Wojakowska; Grzegorz Mazur; Joanna Smardz; Mieszko Wieckiewicz, https://www.ncbi.nlm.nih.gov/pmc/articles/PMC6832407/

"Gender differences in severity of desaturation events following hypopnea and obstructive apnea events in adults during sleep," Antti Kulkas; Brett Duce; Timo Leppänen; Craig Hukins; Juha Töyräs, https://pubmed.ncbi.nlm.nih.gov/28745298/

"Can you really catch up on sleep?," Staff writer, https://www.ahchealthenews.com/2021/07/28/weekend-catch-up-on-sleep/

General

"Burden of disease sleep apnea," WHO / summary, https://www.thelancet.com/journals/lanres/article/PIIS2213-2600(19)30198-5/fulltext

"1 in 3 adults don't get enough sleep," https://www.cdc.gov/media/releases/2016/p0215-enough-sleep.html#print

"Sleep Disordered Breathing: Why Breathing Gets Interrupted During Sleep," Mark Burhenne, https://askthedentist.com/sleep-disordered-breathing/

Anders Olsson, https://www.consciousbreathing.com/

"The connection between insomnia and dental problems," American Academy of Medical Orthodontics, https://medicalorthodontics.org/dental_articles/the-connection-between-insomnia-and-dental-problems/

"Gastroesophageal Reflux Disease and Tooth Erosion," Sarbin Ranjitkar; John A. Kaidonis; and Roger J. Smales, https://www.ncbi.nlm.nih.gov/pmc/articles/PMC3238367/pdf/IJD2012-479850.pdf

"What Are Sleep Deprivation and Deficiency?," https://www.nhlbi.nih.gov/health/sleep-deprivation, https://www.nhlbi.nih.gov/health/sleep-deprivation

"National Sleep Foundation's sleep time duration recommendations: methodology and results summary," Max Hirshkowitz PhD, Kaitlyn Whiton MHS, Steven M. Albert PhD, https://www.sciencedirect.com/science/article/abs/pii/S2352721815000157

"The impact of sleep deprivation on food desire in the human brain," https://www.ncbi.nlm.nih.gov/pmc/articles/PMC3763921/

"What Are Sleep Deprivation and Deficiency?," NIH, https://www.nhlbi.nih.gov/health/sleep-deprivation

"Sympathetic Nervous System (SNS)," Cleveland Clinic, https://my.clevelandclinic.org/health/body/23262-sympathetic-nervous-system-sns-fight-or-flight

"Why Do People Snore?," Johns Hopkins, https://www.hopkinsmedicine.org/health/wellness-and-prevention/why-do-people-snore-answers-for-better-health

"Snoring," Cleveland Clinic, https://my.clevelandclinic.org/health/diseases/15580-snoring

"The Stages of Snoring," Sharon J Borrow, Sleep Laboratory Scientist, St George's Hospital, London, https://britishsnoring.co.uk/stages_of_snoring.php

"We Haven't Connected All the Dots Between Bruxism and Sleep Apnea," C.A. Wolski, https://sleepreviewmag.com/sleep-disorders/movement-disorders/sleep-bruxism/bruxism-sleep-apnea-connection/

"Estimation of the global prevalence and burden of obstructive sleep apnoea: a literature-based analysis," Adam V Benjafield, PhD, https://www.thelancet.com/journals/lanres/article/PIIS2213-2600(19)30198-5/fulltext

"Multinight Prevalence, Variability, and Diagnostic Misclassification of Obstructive Sleep Apnea," Bastien Lechat; Ganesh Naik, https://www.atsjournals.org/doi/10.1164/rccm.202107-1761OC

"Prevalence of sleep bruxism and its association with obstructive sleep apnea in adult patients: a retrospective polysomnographic investigation," Madeleine Wan Yong Tan; Adrian U-Jin Yap; Ai Ping Chua; Johnny Chiew Meng Wong; Maria Victoria Jane Parot; Keson Beng Choon Tan, https://pubmed.ncbi.nlm.nih.gov/30371687/

"Can you really catch up on sleep over the weekend?," https://www.ahchealthenews.com/2021/07/28/weekend-catch-up-on-sleep/

"Orthognathic Surgery: General Considerations," David Y. Khechoyan, MD, https://www.ncbi.nlm.nih.gov/pmc/articles/PMC3805731/

"Mini-implant assisted rapid palatal expansion (MARPE) effects on adult obstructive sleep apnea (OSA) and quality of life: a multi-center prospective controlled trial," Daniel Paludo Brunetto, Christoph E Moschik, Ramon Dominguez-Mompell, Eliza Jaria, Eduardo Franzotti Sant'Anna, Won Moon, https://www.ncbi.nlm.nih.gov/pmc/articles/PMC8804045/pdf/40510_2021_Article_397.pdf

Podcasts/YouTube

"Dru Purohit Podcast, Dhru Purohit (#62) Secret to better sleep with Mark Burhenne DDS," https://dhrupurohit.com/bb-ep62/#ql-video

"How to sleep like your relationship depends on it, Wendy Troxel | TEDxManhattanBeach," https://www.youtube.com/watch?v=U7ntoFtZK6A

"Why do we sleep?," Russel Foster, https://www.ted.com/talks/russell_foster_why_do_we_sleep

"What would happen if you didn't sleep?," Claudia Aguirre TED ed, What would happen if you didn't sleep?

"Want To Be Extraordinary? Start With a Straw," Mark Burhenne DDS, Mark Burhenne | TEDxMontaVistaHighSchool, https://www.youtube.com/watch?v=wdzzvhB5rhg

"Sleep Paradox," Mark Burhenne DDS, https://www.youtube.com/watch?v=D_ATJ9DLPxc

"Mouth Breathing & Mouth Taping," Mark Burhenne DDS on High intensity health, https://www.youtube.com/watch?v=z3lCxl75owQ

"Sleep Is your superpower," Matthew Walker PhD, https://www.ted.com/talks/matt_walker_sleep_is_your_superpower

"A walk through sleep stages," Matthew Walker PhD, https://www.ted.com/talks/matt_walker_a_walk_through_the_stages_of_sleep

"How sleep affects your emotions," Matthew Walker PhD, https://www.ted.com/talks/matt_walker_how_sleep_affects_your_emotions

"Hacking your memory," Matthew Walker PhD, https://www.ted.com/talks/matt_walker_hacking_your_memory_with_sleep

"How much sleep do you really need?," Matthew Walker PhD, https://www.ted.com/talks/matt_walker_how_much_sleep_do_you_really_need

"8 Hours Sleep Paradox," Mark Burhenne, https://www.youtube.com/watch?v=D_ATJ9DLPxc

Websites
Inspire Sleep Apnea Therapy, https://www.inspiresleep.com/path-to-inspire/

https://www.sleepfoundation.org/sleep-deprivation

https://www.aadsm.org

CHAPTER 6: HOW TO BREATHE EASY

Breathing Habits
Breath, James Nestor, Riverhead Books, 2020

"Breathing," Canadian Lung Association, https://www.lung.ca/lung-health/lung-info/breathing

"The effect of nasal and oral breathing on airway collapsibility in patients with obstructive sleep apnea: Computational fluid dynamics analyses," Masaaki Suzukil, Tadashi Tanuma, https://www.ncbi.nlm.nih.gov/pmc/articles/PMC7153879/

"How does open-mouth breathing influence upper airway anatomy?," Seung Hoon Lee , Ji Ho Choi, Chol Shin, Heung Man Lee, Soon Young Kwon, Sang Hag Lee, https://pubmed.ncbi.nlm.nih.gov/17464234/

"Sudarshan kriya yoga: Breathing for health," Sameer A Zope, Rakesh A Zope, https://www.ncbi.nlm.nih.gov/pmc/articles/PMC3573542/pdf/IJY-6-4.pdf

"Learning diaphragmatic breathing," Harvard Medical School, https://www.health.harvard.edu/healthbeat/learning-diaphragmatic-breathing

NO
"Nitric Oxide and the Paranasal Sinuses," Jon O. Lundburg, https://pubmed.ncbi.nlm.nih.gov/18951492/

"Nitric oxide: what's new to NO?," Kedar Ghimire, Helene M. Altmann, Adam C. Straub, and Jeffrey S. Isenberg, https://pubmed.ncbi.nlm.nih.gov/27974299/

"5 Ways to Increase Nitric Oxide Naturally," By Gavin Van De Walle, MS, RD — Medically reviewed by Amy Richter, RD, Nutrition, https://www.healthline.com/nutrition/how-to-increase-nitric-oxide#limit-mouthwash

"NO-Rich Diet for Lifestyle-Related Diseases," Jun Kobayashi, Kazuo Ohtake, and Hiroyuki Uchida, https://www.ncbi.nlm.nih.gov/pmc/articles/PMC4488823/pdf/nutrients-07-04911.pdf

"Dr Mercola's Nitric Oxide Release," Dr Mercola, https://youtu.be/qEui9ImJail?si=L-DmMrUXFXPAgDx0

Tongue
"The anatomical relationships of the tongue with the body system," Brun Bordoni, Bruno Morabito, Roberto Mitrano, Marta Simonelli, Anastasia Toccafondi, https://www.ncbi.nlm.nih.gov/pmc/articles/PMC6390887/

"The assessment of resting tongue posture in different sagittal skeletal patterns," Farheen Fatima, Mubassar Fida, https://www.ncbi.nlm.nih.gov/pmc/articles/PMC6677336/pdf/2176-9451-dpjo-24-03-55.pdf

"What You Need to Know About Proper Tongue Posture," Medically reviewed by J. Keith Fisher, MD— By Jandra Sutton on July 17, 2019, https://www.healthline.com/health/tongue-posture

"Effects of tongue position on mandibular muscle activity and heart rate function," John E. Schmidt, PhD, Charles R. Carlson, PhD, Andrew R. Usery, MD, and Alexandre S. Quevedo, DDS, PhD, http://www.kidstowndentist.com/wp-content/uploads/2015/11/TREATMENT-INFORMATION-Tongue_position_and_muscle_activity.pdf

Conscious Breathing
Conscious Breathing, Anders Olsson, Sorena AB, 2014

Posture
"TREMENDOUS BENEFITS of NOSE Breathing explained by Orthodontist Dr. Ted Belfor" | TAKE A DEEP BREATH, Theodore Belfor, https://www.youtube.com/watch?v=-gBrmHkkooM&t=2068s

"Oral Posture: The Adult Palate and Airway Connection," Steve Lin interviewing Theodore Belfor, https://www.facebook.com/DrStevenLin/videos/291009232373439/

"Posture: The Key to Good Health | Annette Verpillot | TEDxMontrealWomen," Annette Verpillot, https://www.youtube.com/watch?v=S3qdSo8z0Is

Jaws: The story of a Hidden Epidemic, Dr. Sandra Kahn DDS DMD and Paul R. Ehrlich PhD Stanford University Press, 2018

General
"Beneficial effects of UV radiation other than via vitamin D production," Asta Juzeniene & Johan Moan, https://www.tandfonline.com/doi/epdf/10.4161/derm.20013

"The Impact of Mouth-Taping in Mouth-Breathers with Mild Obstructive Sleep Apnea: A Preliminary Study," Yi-Chieh Lee, Chun-Ting Lu, Wen-Nuan Cheng, Hsueh-Yu Li, https://pubmed.ncbi.nlm.nih.gov/36141367/

"Impact of airway dysfunction on dental health," Juliette Tamkin, https://www.ncbi.nlm.nih.gov/pmc/articles/PMC6986941/

Books
Shut your Mouth and Save your Life, George Catlin, https://www.consciousbreathing.com/articles/shut-your-mouth-save-your-life/

Oxygen Advantage, Patrick McKeown, William Morrow, 215

Close Your Mouth – Buteyko Breathing Clinic Self-help Manual, Patrick McKeown, Asthma Care

Breathing Cure, Patrick McKeown, Humanix Books, 2021

The Wim Hof Method, Wim Hof, Sounds True, 2020

Podcasts/YouTube
"The Adult Palate and Airway Connection," Theodore Belfor, https://drtheodorebelfor.com/videos-2/

"Change Your Breath, Change Your Life," Lucas Rockwood, TEDxBarcelona, https://www.youtube.com/watch?v=_QTJOAI0UoU

"Breathe to Heal," Max Strom, TEDxCapeMay, https://www.youtube.com/watch?v=4Lb5L-VEm34

"How breathing and metabolism are interconnected," Ruben Meerman, TEDxBundaberg, https://www.youtube.com/watch?v=nM-ySWylD9o&t=22s

"How to breathe," Belisa Vranich, TEDxManhattanBeach, https://www.youtube.com/watch?v=1sgb2cUqFiY

"The Lost Art of Breathing," James Nestor and Mark Burhenne, https://www.youtube.com/watch?v=VbAEm6-bgGI

CHAPTER 7: GET UP AND GET MOVING

Moving Habits

"Movement as Medicine | TEDxRaleigh,"
Mike Young, https://www.youtube.com/watch?v=jx3EeMaKMJs&list=PLF73236Bj
g_QBY-bPuGZnSn4EMGJ2osQt&index=1&t=194s

"How stress affects your health," American Psychology Association, https://www.apa.org/topics/stress/health

"Stress," APA.org, apa.org https://www.apa.org/topics/stress

"Stress," Adapted from the APA Dictionary of Psychology, https://www.apa.org/topics/stress

"Stress won't go away? Maybe you are suffering from chronic stress," https://www.apa.org/topics/stress/chronic

"Physical Activity Guidelines for Americans," posted on June 27, 2023, by ODPHP, https://health.gov/our-work/nutrition-physical-activity/physical-activity-guidelines

The Joy of Movement: How exercise helps us find happiness, hope, connection, and courage, Kelly McGonigal, Avery, 2021

"Benefits of Physical Activity," CDC, https://www.cdc.gov/physicalactivity/basics/pa-health/index.htm#brain-health

"Stanford Psychologist Reveals How Movement Can Transform Your Life," Kelly McGonigal, https://www.youtube.com/watch?v=IxNlS1W5rg8&t=4s

Digestion

"4 Positive Effects of Exercise on the Digestive System," reviewed Lisa Maloney, CPT author Caroline Haley, https://www.livestrong.com/article/356356-immediate-effects-of-exercise-in-the-digestive-system/

"Exercise Modifies the Gut Microbiota with Positive Health Effects," Vincenzo Monda, Ines Villano, Antonietta Messina, Anna Valenzano, Teresa Esposito, Fiorenzo Moscatelli, Andrea Viggiano, Giuseppe Cibelli, Sergio Chieffi, Marcellino Monda, and Giovanni Messina, https://www.ncbi.nlm.nih.gov/pmc/articles/PMC5357536/

"How the Digestive System & Muscular System Work in Conjunction During Digestion," Kirstin Hendrickson, https://www.livestrong.com/article/262818-how-the-digestive-system-muscular-system-work-in-conjunction-during-digestion/

"Physical Activity and Constipation in Hong Kong Adolescents," Rong Huang, Sai-Yin Ho, Wing-Sze Lo, Tai-Hing Lam, https://www.ncbi.nlm.nih.gov/pmc/articles/PMC3938666/pdf/pone.0090193.pdf

"Why exercise is good for your digestive system," Jo Waters, https://www.healthspan.co.uk/advice/why-exercise-is-good-for-your-digestive-system

Brain

Real Happy Pill: Power Up Your Brain by Moving Your Body, Anders Hansen, Skyhorse Publishing, 2017

"Why the Brain is Built for Movement | TEDxUmeå," Anders Hansen, https://www.youtube.com/watch?v=a9p3Z7L0f0U&t=169s

"How do cognitively stimulating activities affect cognition and the brain throughout life?," Mara Mather, https://www.ncbi.nlm.nih.gov/pmc/articles/PMC7831356/

"World Wide Fingers will advance dementia prevention," Miia Kivipelto, Francesca Mangialasche, Tiia Ngandu, https://www.thelancet.com/journals/laneur/article/PIIS1474-4422(17)30431-3/fulltext

Oral Health

"The association between dental caries and physical activity, physical fitness, and background factors among Finnish male conscripts," Huttunen M, Kämppi A, Soudunsaari A, Päkkilä J, Tjäderhane L, Laitala ML, Anttonen V, Patinen P, Tanner T., https://www.ncbi.nlm.nih.gov/pmc/articles/PMC9810556/pdf/10266_2022_Article_717.pdf

"The impact of oral health on physical fitness: A systematic review," Taufan Bramantoro, Ninuk Hariyani, Dini Setyowati, Bambang Purwanto, https://www.ncbi.nlm.nih.gov/pmc/articles/PMC7182722/pdf/main.pdf

"Physical Activity Reduces the Prevalence of Periodontal Disease:Systematic Review and Meta Analysis," Railson de Oliveira Ferreira, Marcio Gonçalves Corrêa, https://pubmed.ncbi.nlm.nih.gov/30949062/

"The association of sedentary behaviour and physical activity with periodontal disease in NHANES 2011–2012," Maha Almohamad, Elizabeth Krall Kaye, Dania Mofleh, Nicole L. Spartano, https://onlinelibrary.wiley.com/doi/abs/10.1111/jcpe.13669

"Why is exercise important to dentistry?," Rishiniy Pushparatnam, https://www.nature.com/articles/s41407-021-0526-y

"Exercise and oral health: Yes – there is a connection," DrTung's, https://drtungs.com/blog/exercise-and-oral-health-yes-there-is-a-connection-n84#fn1

"The Crazy Way Yoga Can Save Your Dental Health & Correct Your Jawline," Liz Greene, https://www.peacefuldumpling.com/yoga-dental-health

Sleep

"Exercising for Better Sleep," Charlene Gamaldo, M.D. interviewed, https://www.hopkinsmedicine.org/health/wellness-and-prevention/exercising-for-better-sleep

"Exercise and Sleep," Dr. Abhinav Singh, https://www.sleepfoundation.org/physical-activity/exercise-and-sleep

"Sleep and exercise: A reciprocal issue?," Pierrick J Arnal, Damien Leger, https://www.researchgate.net/profile/Pierrick-Arnal/publication/264085860_Sleep_and_exercise_A_reciprocal_issue/links/59e6931aaca2721fc227ae16/Sleep-and-exercise-A-reciprocal-issue.pdf

Mood

"How to Hack Your Hormones for a Better Mood," Medically reviewed by Vara Saripalli, Psy.D. — Crystal Raypole — Updated on Jul 26, 2022, https://www.healthline.com/health/happy-hormone

"Moving improves your mood," Sr Chatterjee and Dr Kelly Gonicgal April 2021, https://shows.acast.com/feelbetterlivemore/episodes/-109discoverthejoyofmovementwithdrkellymcgonigal

"What Exactly Is a Runner's High?," reviewed by Daniel Bubnis, M.S., NASM-CPT, NASE Level II-CSS, Fitness By Kimberly Holland on October 13, 2020, https://www.healthline.com/health/runners-high#definition

IBS
"Irritable bowel syndrome and physical activity," Elisabet Johannesson, https://gupea.ub.gu.se/handle/2077/54963

Oral Health
"Physical Activity Reduces the Prevalence of Periodontal Disease: Systematic Review and Meta-Analysis," Railson de Oliveira Ferreira, Marcio Gonçalves Correa, https://www.frontiersin.org/articles/10.3389/fphys.2019.00234/full

"Why exercise is important for dentistry," Rishiniy Pushparatnam, https://www.nature.com/articles/s41407-021-0526-y.pdf

"Association between Psychological Stress and Periodontitis: A Systematic Review," Micaele M L Castro, Railson de O Ferreira, https://pubmed.ncbi.nlm.nih.gov/32069501/

"Oral health-related behaviours reported by elite and professional athletes," Julie Gallagher, Paul Ashley, Aviva Petrie, Ian Needleman, https://www.nature.com/articles/s41415-019-0617-8

Modulation of oral microbiota: A new frontier in exercise supplementation, Raul Bescos, Zoe L.S. Brookes, Louise A. Belfield, Manuel Fernandez-Sanjurjo, Patricia Casas-Agustench, https://www.sciencedirect.com/science/article/abs/pii/S2213434420300554

Sports Drinks
"Sports and Energy Drink Consumption, Oral Health Problems and Performance Impact among Elite Athletes," Kamran Khan, Abdul Qadir, Gina Trakman, Tariq Aziz, Maria Ishaq Khattak, Ghulam Nabi, Metab Alharbi, Abdulrahman Alshammari, and Muhammad Shahzad, https://www.ncbi.nlm.nih.gov/pmc/articles/PMC9738880/

"Energy Drink Consumption: Beneficial and Adverse Health Effects," Ahmed Abdulrahman Alsunni, MBBS, PhD, https://www.ncbi.nlm.nih.gov/pmc/articles/PMC4682602/

"Modulation of oral microbiota: A new frontier in exercise supplementation," Raul Bescos, Zoe L.S. Brookes, Louise A. Belfield, Manuel Fernandez-Sanjurjo, Patricia Casas-Agustench, https://www.sciencedirect.com/science/article/abs/pii/S2213434420300554

"Exercise improves oral microbiome health," Bio-Practica, https://biopractica.com.au/exercise-improves-oral-microbiome-health/

"Should You Drink Sports Drinks Instead of Water?," Grant Tinsley, Ph.D., CSCS,*D, CISSN, https://www.healthline.com/nutrition/sports-drinks

Walking
"Steve Jobs Loved Walking Meetings. New Research Shows Why He Was Right," Minda Zetlin, https://www.inc.com/minda-zetlin/steve-jobs-walking-meetings-effectiveness-university-hong-kong-experiment-miao-cheng.html

"Here is why Steve Jobs loved to walk and so should you," Johnny Evans, https://www.applemust.com/here-is-why-apples-steve-jobs-loved-to-walk-and-so-should-you/

Connecting with Nature
"How might contact with nature promote human health? Promising mechanisms and a possible central pathway," Ming Kuo, https://www.ncbi.nlm.nih.gov/pmc/articles/PMC4548093/pdf/fpsyg-06-01093.pdf

"What Does Recharge Your Body and Brain Mean," By The fit Team, https://fit.sanfordhealth.org/blog/why-does-recharging-matter

"How to Meditate," Brahma Kumaris, https://www.brahmakumaris.org/meditation/how-to-meditate

Books
The 28-Day Program to Create a Healthy Mouth, Reduce Inflammation and Prevent Disease Throughout the Body, Gerald P. Curatola DDS Center Street, 2017

Exercised, Daniel Lieberman, Penguin UK, 2021

Podcasts/YouTube
"Harvard Professor Reveals How to never be lazy again With Exercise!," Daniel Lieberman interview by Dr Rangan Chatterjee, https://www.youtube.com/watch?v=WWxM_gaVBzE&t=253s

"How to make stress your friend," Kelly McGonigal, https://www.ted.com/talks/kelly_mcgonigal_how_to_make_stress_your_friend/comments

Made in United States
Troutdale, OR
02/27/2024

17996388R00100